Diet Low Carb and Intermittent Fasting

For beginners

Author

Tamara M. Crosby

Introduction

You won't overeat if you have a high protein diet. It won't help you reduce fat or carbohydrates, but it's a safe and efficient alternative. When you eat less without considering your diet, you risk losing critical vitamins and minerals. Muscle spasms and weariness, mental fogginess and hunger, emotional melancholy, irritability, and sleeplessness, as well as a loss of essential minerals and vitamins, might all result from this.

It is possible to lose not just weight but also muscle mass.

The low-carb keto diet enables you to cut down on carbohydrates and calories while still nourishing your body with high-quality oils that help you lose weight without the negative side effects.

It's not a new fad to fast for short periods of time. Since the beginning, it has been aroused. You may fast and lose weight in whatever way you desire. This cookbook includes ketogenic diet recipes to help you lose weight quickly.

Intermittent fasting has grown in popularity in recent years due to its ability to improve nutrient absorption rates. Intermittent fasting is also popular since it doesn't need you to radically alter the sort of food you eat, when you eat it, or how many calories you consume in a 24-hour period. The most common kind of intermittent fasting is eating just two meals each day, rather than the typical three. Intermittent fasting has a wide range of possibilities.

Make use of the ketogenic diet.

For those who have problems keeping to tight diets, the intermittent fasting diet is a good option. There are just a few things that need to be changed. It's easy to stick to for a long time, but it's also effective enough to give the results that keep people engaged long after the novelty of the new eating pattern has worn off.

Intermittent fasting is one of the most effective ways to do so. When you're fasting, your body behaves differently than when you're fed. When your body actively absorbs and digests food, it is said to be active absorption and digestion. This may happen anywhere between 5 and 5 minutes after eating. Depending on how complicated the dish is, it may take anywhere from three to five hours.

When you're hungry, your body creates more insulin, making fat burning more challenging. Insulin levels gradually return to normal when digestion is completed. Between fed and fasted stages, this is known as the buffer state. It might take anywhere between 8 and 12 hours to complete.

When your insulin levels return to normal after a fast, you're in the fasted state. This is when your body is at its most capable of metabolizing fat. As a result, many individuals are unable to effectively burn fat. They seldom go more than eight hours without feeding, and they're much less likely to go longer than twelve hours.

I hope you enjoy and learn from each chapter. Intermittent fasting and ketogenic meals are combined in the ketogenic diet plan. There are enough recipes to cook meals, snacks, breakfast, lunch, and supper for seven days. The Meal Plan for 7 Days will provide you flexibility after you've calculated your calorie allowance.

Chapter 1: The Ketogenic Diet Plan Details

It's important to understand the history of the ketogenic diet before embarking on your intermittent fasting adventure. This isn't a whole new way of eating.

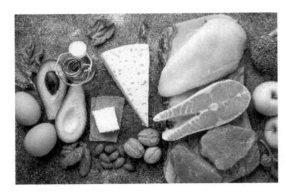

The Keto Diet's History

Ketogenic diets have been around since the dawn of mankind. Bernard McFadden, also known as Bernarr Macfadden, recommended fasting as a form of treatment in order to recover your health. One of McFadden's pupils attempted to cure epilepsy using the same way. Fasting and a sugar-free, starch-free diet were found to be effective in treating epileptic patients, according to the New York Medical Journal in 1912.

In 1921, endocrinologist Rollin Woodyatt discovered the three ketone molecules generated by the liver. Bhydroxybutyrate (acetone), acetone, and acetoacetate were the water-soluble chemicals. Because of a high-fat, low-carbohydrate diet, this happened.

Russell Wilder, a Mayo Clinic physician, gained notoriety in 1921 for his ketogenic diet, which was eventually used as part of an epileptic treatment strategy. The program piqued his curiosity since he suffers from epilepsy. It was also recognized for its other properties, including weight reduction and the treatment of other diseases.

By following these rules, you may start the process of putting your body into ketosis. It's a natural healing process, despite its complexity. Your body will change its metabolism to burn ketones rather than glucose. Fruits, starches, sugars, cereals, and other foods all contain sugar or glucose. In the absence of glucose, your body will burn stored fat.

Find out what works best for you when it comes to a keto diet.

Glucose is most likely your "fuel," which is subsequently converted to dietary energy. The remaining glucose is converted to fat and stored in your body for later use.

The keto diet will be lessened when your body starts to consume stored glucose. After that, your body will start to burn the fat you've accumulated as fuel. Starting with 5% carbohydrates, 75% fats, 20% protein, and 20% calories each day, this new strategy will gradually increase. Calorie counting isn't necessary at all.

presently. Because it's just utilized as a starting point, this is the case. Glucose deficit isn't to blame for these two stages:

Glycogenesis' Stages: Glycogen forms when glucose levels are too high. This is the energy stored in the liver and muscles as glycogen. According to research, you can only conserve roughly half of the energy you consume each day by using glycogen.

Lipogenesis Stages: Any remaining glycogen is stored and transformed to fat.

Similarly to when you sleep, your body will not have any more meals. In order to produce ketones, your body must burn fat. Fats will be broken down into fatty acids by the ketones. They are subsequently oxidized via beta-oxidation in the liver and expelled. When you don't have enough glucose or glycogen, ketosis kicks in, and your body turns to stored/consumed fat for fuel.

At "ketocalculator.ankerl.com," you may use the Internet to find a keto calculator. Begin by making it a habit to check your levels whenever you need to know what nutrients your body requires throughout your diet. Your personal details, such as height and weight, will be kept on file. All of your math may be done using the Internet calculator.

When glycerol and fatty acid molecules are freed, the ketogenesis process commences. The result is acetoacetate. Acetoacetate may produce two kinds of ketone units:

Acetone is mostly eliminated as waste, however it may also be converted to glucose via metabolism. This is why people on the ketogenic diet have a particular odor to their breath.

After you've been on the keto diet for a while, your muscles will convert acetoacetate into beta-hydroxybutyrate, which will feed your brain.

You'll be surprised how adaptive the ketogenic technique is when paired with intermittent fasting. Everyone loses weight in their own unique way, and you may have various objectives.

The easiest method to get started as a novice is to do the following. This is a critical phase in the process. You'll have to make a decision on how you'll carry out your diet plan. This is a very important step that you should address with your physician. These are the four methods for better understanding the different stages of the keto diet:

This ketogenic diet (SKD) is rich in fat, moderate in protein, low in carbohydrates, and high in calories.

The Keto Method #2: At this point, you must adhere to the keto diet's strict guidelines (also known as TKD). When you're active, you should increase your carbohydrate intake.

The cyclical ketogenic diet consists of a five-day ketogenic diet followed by two days of heavy carbohydrate consumption.
The high-protein keto diet (SKD) is comparable to the keto method 4 in every way. You'll eat more protein as a result of this change.

How to Achieve & Maintain Your Diet

These are just a few examples of how any of the diets on the list might help you.

As a starting point, the keto diet emphasizes two crucial factors. A minimum of one meal every day, plus two additional meals per week. Aim for a daily carb intake of no more than 25 grams. This article is meant to assist you in comprehending the overwhelming majority of individuals.

Theory 1: How to Get Started

Step 1: Start the ketogenic diet on a non-stressful week. Step 2: Go through your refrigerator and pantry and clean them out.

Step 3: Fill your refrigerator and pantry with keto-friendly foods.

Step 4: In the mornings, try missing one meal. You may be able to stay up a little later and still enjoy breakfast. (I'll have more to say on Intermittent Fasting in the near future.)

Step 5: Limit your fat and protein intake at first, and don't go over your net carbohydrates.

Step 6: Make a regimen for yourself. 1/2 teaspoon MCT oil or 2 tablespoons coconut oil in a large glass of water

Step 7: Maintain a ketone level diary.

2 Easier Ways to Begin a Ketogenic Diet

If you've tried various low-carb diets or are new to intermittent fasting, try fasting for two days and eating fewer than 20 grams of net carbohydrates each day. This is an excellent method for achieving nutritional ketosis.

Theory 2: Limit sweets, pasta, bread, and other high-carb foods. Sweet potatoes are a better option since they are lower in calories. Limit yourself to 80 grams of sugar every day for a few weeks. Over time, progressively reduce the quantity of net carbohydrates consumed.

Reduce your carb intake in the first step.

Ketosis is achieved with a low-carbohydrate diet. Although sugar/glucose is your cells' principal source of energy, most cells can also run on ketones and fatty acids.

When you eat less carbs, your insulin hormone levels fall. This permits fatty acids from your fat reserve to be released.

Net carbohydrates, which are total carbs plus fiber, may need to be reduced to 20 grams per day for certain people. Others can consume twice as much and yet stay in ketosis. For the first two weeks, keep your carbohydrate consumption to 20 grams or fewer. After that, you may unwind and maintain ketosis.

Step 2: Increase your intake of healthy fats in your diet.

Do not be fooled by the old adage that having too much fat is harmful. It is possible to raise your ketone levels by

fats that are good for your health When you mix a low carbohydrate diet with a high fat intake, you'll go into ketosis. When following the ketogenic diet for weight loss, you may acquire 60 to 80 percent of your calories from fat. Fat accounts for 8590 percent of the calories in the conventional epileptic diet.

Because you'll be eating a lot of fat, high-quality food is crucial. Butter, avocado oil, and lard are three healthy fats that may be utilized in cooking. While many high-fat meals have low carbohydrate content, it's still necessary to keep track of them to stay in ketosis. You should consume at least 60% of your calories from fat to enhance your ketone levels. Animal and plant sources are also available.

Step 3: Continue to eat a healthy amount of protein.

Amino acids that can be utilized to produce new glucose must be provided to your liver (gluconeogenesis). Your liver produces glucose to power cells and organs that can't utilize ketones. Red blood cells, kidneys, brain, and liver are among the organs affected.

Protein may assist maintain muscle mass when carb consumption is restricted. This is particularly true while attempting to lose weight. Protein consumption for every pound of lean body mass should be between 0.55-0.77 grams, according to research. This will help you maintain muscle mass while also improving your athletic abilities.

It's as simple as that: too much protein suppresses ketone production while also causing muscle mass loss. Step 4: Consume Coconut Oil as Part of Your Keto Diet

Patients with neurological illnesses like Alzheimer's disease may also utilize oil to boost their ketone levels.

MCTs (medium-chain triglycerides) are abundant in coconut oil, and they help to speed up the ketosis process. MCTs are rapidly absorbed and transported to the liver, where they may be utilized for energy right away. Ketones are produced as a consequence of this. Oil contains these fats, with lauric acid accounting for half of them. According to study, a larger proportion of coconut oil may result in long-term ketosis. Because it is digested more slowly than other MCTs, it has this effect.

Because coconut oil might induce diarrhea and stomach cramps, it's best to introduce it to your diet gradually. Start with a teaspoon of coconut oil every day and gradually increase to two or three teaspoons every other day after a week.

Step 5: Check Ketone Levels and Make Diet Adjustments

Maintaining ketosis is a process that is unique to each individual. Make certain you're on track to meet your objectives. Acetone and acetoacetate levels in the blood, breath, urine, and skin may all be measured.

A Ketonix meter may be used to track your breathing. Inhaling turns on the meter. The data will be shown on a specific color coded display that shows your ketosis levels.

Ketones may be measured with a blood ketone tester, which looks like a glucose monitor. Put a drop of blood on a test strip and then into your meter. This will reveal your blood's beta-hydroxybutyrate level. Sadly, these strips may be extremely costly. ketosis levels at the moment

Detect acetoacetates in your urine. To modify the color of the strip, dip it into urine. The different hues of pink and purple represent different amounts of ketones. The test strip darkens as the level rises. They're also rather inexpensive. It's better to do your test first thing in the morning following a ketogenic supper the night before.

To remain in ketosis, you may utilize these strategies to see whether you need to adjust your diet.
What Should You Do If You Make a Mistake?
Returning to ketosis is complicated by a number of variables. Your success will be influenced by the following factors:
Your metabolic rate, hormone profile, and other factors all play a role in your overall health. To get out of ketosis, what did you eat? Before the lapse, how long had you been in ketosis?
How much muscle mass you have and how often you workout are two factors to consider.

Most individuals will be in ketosis again after one to three days. Fasting, MCT oil, and ketones may all help to speed things up. If you're looking to go back into ketosis after a carb binge, you'll need to do the following:

Protein consumption should be restricted.
Reduce your sugar and carb intake as soon as possible.

Keep an eye on your ketone levels to evaluate which hypothesis works best for you.

Ketogenic Diet Advantages

You haven't had anything to eat for quite some time. Carbohydrates are not as long-lasting as fat. You'll have to wait longer to feel satiated after eating. The "full state" will remain longer if you eat meals high in carbohydrates.

Other advantages of the ketogenic diet include: It may aid in the treatment of the following conditions:

The ketogenic diet has been shown to reduce seizures in children who have followed it effectively. The therapeutic keto diet for epilepsy limits carb consumption to fewer than 15 grams per day in order to elevate ketone levels even further. Without the guidance of a physician, you should not try to attain these levels.

It is possible to lose weight rapidly if you are fat or overweight. It's critical to stick to the keto diet plan in order to achieve your weight-loss goals.

Improvements in pre-diabetes and diabetes: The keto diet will help you lose weight while also addressing metabolic syndrome, type 2 diabetes, and prediabetes.

Eliminating grains from your diet reduces joint pain and stiffness significantly. Chronic pain and other chronic ailments are thought to be caused by grain-based meals.

Your brain is 60% fat, which limits your ability to think critically. If you consume a lot of high-fat foods, you could feel confused. It may benefit from ketosis to help it reach its full potential and perform optimally.

Many forms of cancer and slow growths are treated with the keto diet.

Alzheimer's disease progresses more slowly in Alzheimer's patients: The keto diet may help to slow down the growth of the illness and lessen symptoms.
Blood pressure levels are lower: While you're on the plan, talk to your doctor about reducing your medications. If you don't consume enough carbohydrates, you may feel dizzy.

It is possible to enhance your cholesterol profile: High cholesterol and triglyceride levels are often linked to arterial plaque formation. These levels have been reported to rise while following a ketogenic diet.

Gum Disease and Tooth Decay Issues Have Been Resolved Your gum troubles should go away after three months if you stick to the regimen. Ketosis's Side Effects
There are likely to be several concerns when you begin your new diet. These are only a few examples to assist you figure out how to handle them.

Dehydration or a lack of salt consumption might cause heart palpitations. You may add additional carbs to your diet plan, but if you don't feel better after that, you should seek emergency medical attention.

Your diet has drastically altered in the last 24 hours, causing digestive troubles. It's common to have constipation and diarrhea when you first start the keto diet. Because dehydration may cause constipation, you should drink plenty of water. Low-carbohydrate diets are part of the issue. Because everyone is different, increasing your fiber intake will depend on the foods you consume. You may cut down on new foods until you're in the transitional period of ketosis. Over time, the symptoms should fade.

Beneficial microorganisms in your stomach may be in short supply. Consume fermented foods to boost your probiotic levels and aid your digestion. Enzymes, B vitamins, and omega 3 fatty acids may all help. Eat the correct veggies and season your diet with a little of salt to help you move about more easily. If everything else fails, take Milk of Magnesia.

Leg Cramps: When the keto diet plan alterations are adopted, a lack of magnesium (a mineral) might cause discomfort. Because of the loss of minerals during urine, you may have leg cramps.

Ketosis and sleep patterns: If you fasted for more than eight hours, your body will be in ketosis. The ketones may then be burned. If you're new to low-fat or high-carb diets, getting into the proper fat-burning condition takes time. Carbs and glucose are vital to your health. It will have a hard time giving up carbohydrates and will want saturated fats.
Restlessness at night is another negative effect.

Low insulin or serotonin levels may occasionally be treated with supplements. For a fast dose, combine a half-teaspoon of fruit spread and a dark chocolate square. It is conceivable, despite the fact that it may seem ludicrous. The carbohydrates in your DIY cure must still be counted.

Induction The flu is real, and the diet may make you angry, queasy, or perplexed.

After a few days, the symptoms should subside. Half a teaspoon of salt in a glass of water may help relieve adverse effects. For the first week, this may entail repeating the technique once a day. It may take up to 15-20 minutes to begin. Relax, since it'll pass quickly.

Carbohydrates might help you retain more hydration if you're thirsty. Once carbohydrates are removed, water weight is shed. You may compensate for this by increasing your water consumption, since you're probably dehydrated. Because you're storing carbohydrates, you'll need extra water on the ketogenic diet.

If you're dehydrated, your body will utilize stored carbohydrates to rehydrate you. Carbohydrates are gone, and the body is dehydrated. Because the ketogenic state is diuretic, drink plenty of water throughout the day.

Ketosis is indicated by foul urine and high acetone levels. It's very natural for your body to acclimatize to this new situation. There's nothing to worry about.

Dairy and Your Diet: What You Can Eat To Stay In Ketosis

The ketogenic lifestyle necessitates a thorough knowledge of dairy and dairy products. Lactose intolerance may prevent you from following the ketogenic diet. Four ounces per day should be the maximum limit. Choose fermented, keto-friendly dairy products.

The best option is unsweetened almond milk. There's

also flax and hemp milk.

When it comes to butter, ghee, and milk solids, what is the difference? Water, butterfat, and milk solids combine to make butter. Ghee, on the other hand, is a butterfat-based Indian delicacy. Lactose intolerance sufferers should opt for ghee. Ghee also contains medium chain fatty acids, which might aid digestion and strengthen your immune system.

Foodstuffs

You must be cautious while selecting sweeteners since some are higher in carbs than others. The Glycemic Index determines how much blood sugar must rise after consuming a specific food. If it has a zero next to it, it is unlikely to raise your blood glucose levels. This is the insulin concentration at the start of the experiment. According to the GI, this will assist you in selecting the best option for your requirements and preferences:

GI: 0; Stevia (liquid) GI: 0 for aspartame GI: 0 for erythritol Monk GI (Glycemic Index) of fruit: 0. GI: 0 for inulin
GI:13 xylitol
Sucralose is a sugar substitute that is used to sweet (liquid) GI (Gross Domestic Product): GI: 36 Maltitol GI: Saccharin

Sweeteners for Keto Diets: 7 of the Best

From most popular to least popular, these sweeteners are ranked. Consider all of your options before deciding on a sweetener. Although the recipes are adaptable, many of them recommend using a specific product.

Option 1: The best sweetener is Pyure's Organic All Purpose Blend. There is no bitterness in this stevia-based product. This sweetening, baking, and cooking blend of stevia and erythritol is a great alternative. Substitute 1/3 teaspoon Pyure for every teaspoon of sugar. This can be changed to suit your tastes.

Powdered sugar can be made by grinding the sweetener until it is completely dry in your NutriBullet/blender.

Swerve Granular sweetener (option 2) is another excellent option. It's made up of indigestible carbohydrates derived from starchy root vegetables and fruits. If you don't like the taste or texture of stevia, this is a great alternative.

Sugar can be replaced with swerve. For each one, begin with 3/4 teaspoon sugar. Increase the quantity as needed. Swerve

For your baking needs, it also has its own confectioners'/powdered sugar. On the downside, it is more expensive (roughly twice as much as the Pyure) than other similar products. You must decide whether the difference in price is worthwhile.

NOW Foods' Purist sweetener is made entirely of erythritol. The sugar content of the product is roughly 70%. As a result, a little more is required. In place of one teaspoon of sugar, use 1 1/3 to 1 1/2 teaspoons erythritol.

Option 4: Xylitol is a sugar substitute that was recently added to the sugary list. It tastes like sugar and is great for sweetening teriyaki and BBQ sauces.

The Glycemic index (GI) of natural sugar alcohol is 13. This might be for you if you've tried everything else. A minty aftertaste has been reported by some users.

It is commonly found in chewing gum to keep your mouth bacteria in check and improving.
A - which gum can be considered a laxative if consumed in large quantities If you're going to use a lot of it, you'll need a lot of Due to the toxicity of this ouse, it should be handled with care.

Note: Even small amounts are toxic to dogs. Brown sugar is an option on d's list. The sugar content of the stevia mixture is one-to-one. It's best to start with a teaspoon of sugar per teaspoon of sugar. If you're looking for a job, this isn't the best option, according to the ed States.

Alternative to gluten. Ut, vanilla, and chocolate are among the flavors available from Sweet Leaf. It is possible to

To make a sweetened extract, combine all of the ingredients in a blender and process until smooth Stevia Drockly (option 6) However, everyone is different, and some people believe it is a matter of personal preference. To make one teaspoon, only three drops are needed.

sugar.

Choice 7: When making pancakes, it's especially important to use the right syrup. Monkfruit and Erythritol are used in Lakanto's Maple-flavored Sugar-Free Syrup. You can also use Golden Monk Fruit Sweetener as a substitute for brown sugar. Over 1,000 years ago, Buddhist monks gave the fruit the name monk-fruit. It's a cooling agent, so it might not be ideal for your digestive system. Please be cautious when using it in baked goods.

Spices to Avoid

Because many store-bought spices contain sugar, you'll need to learn how to make your own.

Labels must be read. Table salt is preferable to sea salt because it is frequently combined with powdered glucose. Frequently used items include:
Cilantro Black pepper, cayenne pepper, and sea salt are all used in the preparation of basil.
powdered chili

Turmeric is an orange-colored Asian herb that is used in both Ayurvedic and Chinese medicine. Turmeric contains curcumin, an anti-inflammatory compound that aids in blood sugar regulation and insulin receptor function. Turmeric can be used in meats, smoothies, and green drinks. Add the turmeric after the meal is done cooking.

Turmeric also has the following health advantages:

Lowers the level of cholesterol Getting in Shape Alzheimer's disease can be avoided by taking this supplement. Controls diabetes and alleviates arthritis. Digestion is improved.

Fermented foods are good for your digestive system, such as pickles, sauerkraut, and coconut milk kefir. Natural acids can also help to keep blood sugar under control.

Enzymes, probiotics, and other bioactive nutrients help to keep the body in ketosis. All of these are fantastic reasons to consume fermented foods. Fermented foods can aid in the re-establishment of beneficial bacteria in the gastrointestinal tract.

Probiotics: Probiotics can be found in kimchee, Greek yogurt, and kefir. Also available are supplements.

Cinnamon can help you increase the activity of your insulin receptors. Just combine

1/2 teaspoon cinnamon in a shake or other keto dessert This is an ingredient that appears in a lot of keto recipes.

Lime and lemon, both high in citric acid, can help you naturally lower your blood sugar levels. Taking trace minerals in lemon or lime, such as potassium, can help you raise your insulin levels. Your liver function will improve as a result of this. They're good in overcooked meats and green juices, among other things. They can also be added to your salad to help you get into ketosis. Here are a few of the numerous advantages:

Weight-loss-friendly Immune system booster purifier of the blood Lowers fever by balancing pH
Decreases blemishes and wrinkles by flushing out unwanted materials. Infections of the lungs are relieved. Toothache pain is relieved.

ACV (Apple Cider Vinegar): This acetic acid can reduce the amount of carbohydrate in a typical meal by 31%. The glycemic response is reduced. ACV contains enzymes that help with fat and protein metabolism. It can be mixed with 8 ounces of water and 1 to 2 tablespoons vinegar or added straight. Here are just a few of ACV's many advantages:

An excellent source of energy. Improves digestion and aids in weight loss
It boosts your immune system and is great for detoxing. cholesterol levels are reduced
Aids in the relief of muscle aches and pains.
Controls blood sugar and helps with diabetes.

Healthy Fats help to balance your inner body.

The ketogenic diet requires fats to be successful. Although fats are necessary in your diet, you must know which fats are beneficial and which are harmful. Omega-3 and Omega-6 fatty acids should be in balance.

Omega-3 fatty acids are beneficial to your overall health. Salmon, tuna, shellfish, and trout are all excellent choices. If you don't like fish, you can substitute fish oil supplements or krill oil.

Avocado, butter, and coconut oil contain monounsaturated and saturated fats. Also delicious are egg yolks and macadamia nuts. Dressings, sauces, and butter can all be made with these ingredients.
Coconut oil and ghee, for example, are non-hydrogenated oils. They produce more smoke because they produce more

In comparison to other oils, the oil has less oxidation. Just a few examples:

Butter and Oil from Avocados Palm Oil with Red Color
Chicken Fat Mayonnaise (non-hydrogenated lard) (watch the carbs) Avocado oil, coconut oil, and sesame oil are three of the most common oils used in cooking.

Coconut flakes (flaxseed oil)

Macadamia nuts are a kind of tree that grows in the United States.
Macadamia Oil: Macadamia oil has a high smoke point, which is one of its advantages. It has a moderate taste and may be used in mayonnaise as a substitute for olive oil. Extra-Virgin Olive Oil (EVOO) from Olives, with a Note:

Olive oil is one of the earliest edible oils that has ever been discovered. It has been used in cooking since at least 1000 B.C. It was used to anoint priests and monarchs, although it may also be utilized for other purposes. It's adaptable, delicious, and beneficial to your general health.

Olive oil has been demonstrated in studies to preserve your vascular system and reduce LDL cholesterol, which may help avoid cardiovascular disease. Extra-virgin oil has been proven to boost the development of probiotic "Bifido" bacteria strains, which is good for the gut microbiome, according to new study.

Olive oil contains monounsaturated fats, which have been related to improved blood sugar control. Fasting glucose levels are lower, and inflammatory levels are lower.
Extra-virgin oil also resists oxidation better than conventional cooking oils when heated, according to research. High-quality, low-acidity extra-virgin olive oils (EVOO) have a smoky flavor.

410 degrees Fahrenheit Olive oil is more stable than other cooking fats, thus this is greater than what most culinary applications need.

Vegetables

Net Carbs per 100g or 1/2 cup for each one are as follows:

0.2 kg. sprouted Alfalfa seeds 2.05 oz. arugula 1.78 oz. asparagus
3 Beans - Green Snap - 3.6 oz. bamboo shoots

0.63 pounds of beet greens Broccoli with bell peppers (4.04 oz.)
3 Savoy Cabbage

6.78 lb. carrots
Baby carrots (5.34 oz.)

Cauliflower is a vegetable that has a calorie count of 2.97. Celery– 1.37 Chard– 2.14 Chicory greens– 0.7 Chives– 1.85 Coriander– Cilantro Leaves– 0.87 Cucumber– 3.13 Eggplant– 2.88 30.96 oz. garlic Kale – 5.15 Leeks – bulb (+), bottom leaf – 12.35 Ginger root – 15.77

Citronella (lemongrass) 25.31 Lettuce – red leaf – 1.36 Lettuce – crisp-head varieties, such as iceberg 1.77 Brown Mushrooms – 3.7 Mustard Mustard Mustard Mustard Mustard Mustard Mustard Mustard Mustard Mustard Mustard Yellow onions – 7.64 greens – 1.47 4.74 oz. spring onions or scallions
6.65 oz. sweet onion Banana peppers (1.95 oz) Chili peppers - scorching hot - 7.31 Jalapeo peppers (3.7 oz.) 2.94 green sweet peppers
Sweet and red peppers - 3.93 Sweet and yellow peppers (5.42 oz.)

Mushrooms Portabella — 2.57 oz. Radishes – 1.8 8.27 Pumpkin – 6 Kelp - Kelp - Kelp Kelp Kelp Kelp Kelp Kelp Kelp Kel Spirulina is a kind of seaweed that is found in abundance in the Mediterranean.
4.29 oz. shiitake mushrooms 1.43 lbs. spinach

Crookneck Squash — Summer – 2.64 lbs.

Zucchini (Squash) 2.11 Squash - acorn - acorn squash - acorn squash - acorn squash - acorn squash - acorn

Turnips – 4.63 Tomatoes – 2.69 Tomatoes – 2.69 Tomatoes – 2.69 Tomatoes
3.93 pound turnip greens White 2.26 lbs. mushrooms These are also nutritious:
Squash & Parsnips

Zucchini with Peas

Fruits to Choose

This is a half-cup portion of keto fruits (100g): 13.6 apricots (no skin) Bananas (7.5 lbs.) Cantaloupe – 6 Kiwi –
14.2 Oranges – 11.7 Oranges – 23.4 Blackberries – 23.1 Blueberries – 22.1 Cantaloupe – 6 Kiwi – 14.2 Oranges –
11.7 Oranges

11.6 peaches, 19.2 pears

Watermelon 7.1 Pineapple 11 Plums 16.3 Kiwi 15 Pineapple Pineapple Pineapple Pineapple Pineapple Pineapple
Pineapple Pineapple Pineapple Pineapple Pineapple Pine

The following are just a handful of the various Keto diet options:

a squeeze of lemon juice from limes
Strawberries Melon casaba olives that are green Avocados Black Olives With Coconut Rhubarb
Starfruit (Carambola) Gooseberries
Acerola, often called West Indian Cherry, is a fruit native to the Caribbean. Oheloberries Boysenberries Grapefruit
It should be noted that the fruit and vegetable values are simply estimations. For each recipe in this book, these
figures were determined.
Nutritional Supplements
High-quality proteins are emphasized on the keto diet. As a starting point, consider these items:
Thighs, breasts, drumsticks, and ground chicken are among the chicken products available.

Wild-caught fish is preferable. Fresh or canned tuna, trout, salmon, and snapper, as well as cod, mahimahi,
mackerel, cod, halibut, and mahimahi, should all be included in your diet.

Crabs, clams, lobster, oysters, scallops, squid, shrimp, or mussels are some of the shellfish to choose from. Fish:
portioned wild caught salmon in freezer bags Duck, chicken, pheasant, or quail are all available as poultry options.

Ground Turkey and Turkey Breasts

Look for free-range eggs at a local market. Scrambled, fried, boiled, and devil egg sandwiches may be made for every occasion.

Natural peanut butter is a good option, but keep in mind that it contains a lot of carbs and Omega-6 fatty acids. A sensible option is macadamia nut butter.

Meat: Grass-fed meat has a greater fatty acid content, thus it's preferred. Lamb, veal, or goat are the options. Flap steak, sirloin, and chuck roast, as well as lean ground beef, are all options.

Avoid bacon and sausage that has been cured in sugar or has excessive fillers. Pork chops, loins, and ham are all excellent choices. You must, however, be wary of the sugar that has been added.
Venison is a nutritious meat. Macadamia nuts, sesame seeds, flax seeds, chia seeds, and other fresh nuts

You may be asking why carbohydrates and proteins are so crucial when you start ketosis via intermittent fasting. Here's why they're so crucial to your diet:

Protein is a Fat Burner: Studies have revealed that your body cannot utilize or burn fat as quickly as it can use or burn other energy sources. This is due to a deficiency in protein or carbohydrates in your body. Maintaining a proper intake of protein is critical for preserving your lean, calorie-burning muscles.

Protein helps you burn calories by slowing digestion and making it simpler to consume the foods you want. During the initial phase of your diet plan, it's critical that you feel full. Allowing yourself to eat everything you want is not a good idea. Muscle Growth and Repair: On days when you are physically active, you should consume more protein. It's critical to comprehend the carbohydrate, protein, and fat ratios and have a strong understanding of them. You aim to achieve balance, which may be found in a specialized eating plan such as the keto diet.

Carbohydrates

Your body transforms all of the carbohydrates you eat into glucose, which gives you a jolt of energy. Carbs stored in the liver provide around 50-60% of your calories. After then, the glycogen is released as required. Adenosinetriphosphate (ATP) is an energy molecule, and glucose is required for its creation. Glucose is required for your body's regular functions and upkeep. Once the liver has reached its capacity, it will convert any surplus carbs to fat.

Ketosis Support Supplements
On the ketogenic diet, you may receive necessary nutrients in a variety of methods, including:

Many foods contain beta-carotene. Because many of these meals are heavy in carbohydrates, a keto-friendly individual may not be able to consume them all. It's crucial to keep in mind that too much vitamin A may be harmful, so keep that in mind.

Make sure you obtain your beta carotene from natural foods rather than pills. The following is a list of keto-friendly foods that contain beta carotene.

Asparagus Dandelion Greens Broccoli Collard Greens Peppers with Kale and Onions Pumpkin-spinach

The greater the beta carotene content, the more yellow-orange the color. The chlorophyll in lush leaves hides yellow-orange.

Calcium is required for healthy bones, muscular contractions, and blood clotting. You may get your calcium from a variety of sources, including the following:

Non-dairy and dairy milks that are unsweetened and zero carbs Leafy vegetables such as broccoli Calcium supplements, as well as Vitamin D supplements, may be required. Calcium should be consumed by both men and women on a daily basis in the amount of 1000 mg.

Vitamin D is required for hormone and nutrition synthesis in the body. Vitamin D, on the other hand, may be obtained outdoors. Prevent skin cancer by avoiding excessive sun exposure. The D vitamin also aids in the absorption of magnesium, calcium, and other essential minerals. This aids in the development of muscles and the preservation of bone density. Your D vitamin level is comparable to that of around 1/3 of the population of the United States. Take 400 IU per day as suggested and include fatty fish and mushrooms in your diet to enhance your intake. Chlorella is a green algae-based superfood that may help you battle tiredness. It also includes Chlorella Growth Factor, a nutrient with DNA and RNA that aids in energy exchange between cells. Capsules, pills, and powder form of the supplement are all available. You may make a daily drink out of it by mixing it with water, smoothies, or any other liquid.

Spirulina is a chlorella-like blue-green algae. It is a complete protein because it includes all of the required amino acids. It's also high in magnesium, iron, and potassium, as well as other minerals that are good for you. It's well-known for its antioxidant capabilities. It's been shown to help those with high cholesterol and blood pressure. It raises HDL (good cholesterol) while lowering LDL (bad cholesterol) (bad cholesterol). It may be taken as a capsule or as a powder.

Foods to Avoid If You Don't Want to Stay Ketosis

When you follow the ketogenic diet, you have a lot of healthful options.

diet. Unless they've been meticulously organized in a cookbook or other expert sources, you should avoid the following foods.

Sugars added: You should avoid sweets such as honey, maltose, and dextrose. Avoid the following sugars:

Corn syrup (dextrose)

Honey Maltose Fructose

Artificial sweeteners, including saccharin and sucralose, should be avoided.

Regular Dairy Milk: Regular dairy milk has about 13 grams of carbohydrates per cup, therefore it's best to avoid it.

Alcoholic drinks should be used in moderation, with the following exceptions:

Mixers: flavored liquor Beer Dry wine Cocktails: flavored liquor Cocktails: flavored liquor Cocktails: flavored liquor Cocktails: Soda, juice, or syrup are all examples of sugar-based beverages. Some experts believe as well.

acceptability of these spirits:

Check the carb level of vodka, since it is often made from potatoes, rye, and wheat (grain-based). The grains utilized include whiskey, maize, barley, rye, and wheat, all of which contain no carbohydrates or sugar. Choose rums with no added sugar or carbohydrates.

Tequila: The agave plant is where tequila comes from.

Drinking alcohol is not advised. Alcohol, on the other hand, causes your liver to create ketones. Alcohol should be drunk in very tiny doses to prevent any negative health consequences.

Only eat these foods on rare occasions.

These are OK to use on occasion, but they will add additional carbs to your dishes. Here are a few "some-timers" to stay away from:

Agave nectar offers 5 grams of carbohydrates per teaspoon, compared to 4 grams of table sugar.

Peas, lentils, kidney beans, and chickpeas are among the beans and legumes to stay away from. Count the carbohydrates, protein, and fat content if you utilize them.

Corn oil, sunflower oil, almonds, pine nuts, and walnuts are examples of nut or seed-based products that should be watched since they contain high levels of inflammatory Omega-6s.

Cashews and pistachios: These delicious nuts should be consumed with caution due to their high carbohydrate content.
These fats, which also include margarine, have been related to coronary heart disease.
When utilizing vegetable oils like safflower, olive, soybean, or flaxseed, cold-pressed goods should be avoided.

Products made from corn Potatoes and potato-related goods are a staple of the American diet.

Artificial sweeteners may trigger ketosis if you consume a lot of diet Coke. The key is moderation. Artificial sweetness and sugar cravings are linked, according to research. As a result, controlling these beverages is more challenging.

Chapter 2: Intermittent Fasting CombinedWith the Ketogenic Diet Plan

Not everyone is a fan of intermittent fasting. In this chapter, you'll learn how to practice Intermittent Fasting and how to form long-term habits. It's not as necessary to know the precise time you'll fast as it is to speed as long as you can.

The Benefits of Intermittent Fasting

Fasting isn't exactly a new fad. Christianity, Islam, Buddhism, and Islam have all practiced it. Fasting may have been abandoned due to a long period of difficulty to acquire food supplies. It isn't a starvation diet since hunger is defined as a shortage of food that occurs due to circumstances beyond one's control. The first meal of the day is the most significant. Every day begins with breakfast.

If you modify your fasting schedule too often, your hormones will become irregular, making weight loss more difficult. You could have a hard time finding the right meal to break your fast with.

Intermittent fasting is done in a variety of ways, but the core principles remain the same. You may experiment with a few to find which one best suits your needs. It's important not to restrict your calorie intake too soon.

How to Make Your Metabolism Work for You

Even while intermittent fasting requires a lot of effort, there are techniques to speed up the process. To hasten your weight reduction, consume these foods:

Food Groups with a High Protein Content
The digestion of these goods will need extra effort: Eggs nut and seed combinations
Legumes Meat from the sea

The thermomic effect of food (TEF) is what your body need to absorb and digest nutrients from meals. By boosting your protein consumption, you'll feel satiated for longer and be less likely to overeat.

Vitamins and minerals that are required by the body

Zinc, iron, and a sufficient amount of selenium are essential for good health. Low intake of these components has been proven in studies to impair the thyroid gland's ability to produce critical hormones. The metabolism will slow dramatically as a result of this. Fruits, vegetables, and whole grains should all be included in your diet.

seafood as well as meat Consider the following further resources:

Tea: The catechins in tea combine with the caffeine in the tea to help speed up your metabolism. Catechins are a form of natural phenol that belongs to the flavonoids chemical family and act as an antioxidant. With the use of green and oolong tea, you may burn an extra 100 calories each day and boost your metabolism by four to ten percent. Each person who is fasting may have distinct impacts.

Caffeine may help you burn 11 percent more calories by increasing your metabolic rate. According to studies, drinking at least 270 mg of caffeine each day (about three cups of coffee) burns an extra 100 calories every day. If you keep it sugar-free, the rates will undoubtedly help you with intermittent fasting.

Chili Peppers: Capsaicin, a substance present in chili peppers, is a metabolism booster. During your intermittent fasting regimen, the capsaicin will improve your fat and calorie burn. According to twenty studies, you'd burn an additional fifty calories every day. However, the hypothesis is now accepted by all scientists. Enjoy the chili peppers, in either case.

Intermittent Fasting's Fundamental Techniques
Another term for this regimen is the Lean-Gains Method. It's designed to help you lose weight and build muscle. There are some obvious advantages to this sort of fasting. It may be tailored to your specific requirements and works with a range of time frames.
This method enables you to fast for 16 hours and eat for 8 hours each day while being safe.

Men and women will fast for 14 and 16 hours respectively. They may consume a reasonable quantity of calories for the following 8-10 hours after that. People often break up the 8-10 hour period into three smaller meals or have two major meals. This is due to the fact that the majority of individuals eat in a predetermined manner.

According to a research done by the Obesity Society, eating supper before 2:00 p.m. reduces hunger throughout the day. You'll also improve your fat-burning skills. During the fasting phase, you should avoid consuming high-calorie foods like black coffee (with a little cream), water, diet soda, and sugar-free gum. Avoid eating after supper and wait 14 hours before eating again to adhere to this plan.

The Warrior Diet is a 16:8-style diet. It is suggested that you fast for 20 hours every day and then consume one meal for the remaining four hours.

The assumption that people normally feed at night underpins intermittent fasting. By eating at night, the body is better able to absorb nutrients. Fasting in this case, as it occurs throughout the day, may be a bit perplexing.

For a period of 20 hours, you are permitted to have a portion of fruits or vegetables and a little quantity of protein.

This program stimulates the body's natural nervous system, causing it to become more alert and energized. It also boosts fat-burning efficiency. The body can focus on its own recovery and improvement if it eats a large meal every evening. Every evening, it is critical that you begin with vegetables. Following that, you should consume protein, fat, and carbs that are keto-friendly.

Fasting is so popular for two reasons: The first is that fasting allows for small, reasonable snacks. For those who are trying to lose weight, this is a plus. Over the course of the week, the majority of people who try this fasting report a significant increase in energy and fat loss.

It may be difficult to maintain a strict diet for long periods of time. It can also make social interactions more difficult. Some people despise being forced to consume their meals in a specific order. To see if you like it, you can try it out for yourself.

Because you can fast without triggering your hormones or shocking any part of your body, the Crescendo Method is suitable for women. This is a safe program for women, but it does require a 12- to 16-hour fast. You'll be able to savor your meals for up to 8 hours. You could do it on Monday, Wednesday, and Friday, for example. If you've tried and failed with other diets, this might be the right fit for you. After a two-week period, you can add one more day of active fasting.

Eat-Stop-Eat, or the 24-Hour Protocol: You can fast for 24 hours using this technique. This can only be done twice a week, though. Make a decision on a date. Fasting between the hours of 8 a.m. and 8 a.m. is thought to be easier because you'll be sleeping the majority of the time. Ketosis is a metabolic state that occurs naturally in the body. It's critical to stick to a regular or reasonable diet after you've finished fasting and avoid binging for an extended period of time. Fasting or bingeing for long periods of time can be harmful to your body. It's critical to practice moderation and self-control when fasting to get the most out of it.

By reducing 3,500 calories per week, the fast cycle assumes you can lose one pound per week. Fasting for one day might be preferable to losing weight in two short bursts. This fasting plan focuses on resistance weight training for the best results.

Going a day without eating can be difficult. Fasting for longer periods of time and increasing the amount of time are both possible. It's an excellent place to begin. Pick days when you won't be obligated to eat anything. When you know you'll be attending a lunch meeting, it's not a good idea to start a fasting program.

Fatigue, headaches, anger, and anxiety are all common fasting side effects. When you first begin the fast, these side effects can be a problem. These side effects will diminish as your body adjusts to this new cycle.

After a long day of eating healthily, it's natural to want to binge on your first meal. Bingeing is not only bad for your health, but it can also quickly undo all of your hard work from the previous 24 hours. Self-discipline can help you make fasting more worthwhile.

Fat Loss Forever: This type of intermittent fasting incorporates elements from several different styles to create something unique. The good news is that you get a cheat-day every week. That's correct.

After a one-and-a-half-day fast, the rest of the week is divided between 16:8 and 20:4 fasting.

Fasting 16:8 or 20:4 for the rest of the week.

cycle of 24 hours Maintaining as much activity as possible during these days will help to curb your hunger. If you have trouble controlling your hunger on cheat days, intermittent fasting isn't for you. It necessitates a quick and consistent drop from 70 to zero.

It is not advisable to go 36 hours without eating. Fasting requires your body to adjust. It's best to start with intermittent fasting and then progress to Fat Loss Forever once you've eliminated your three-to-four-hour eating habits.

When fasting, always remember to be responsible and not overwork your body.

Alternate-Day Diet - This type of intermittent fasting does not necessitate fasting for long periods of time. Every two days, you should eat. On non-working days, you'll consume only one-fifth of the calories you would on a typical day.

Between 2,000 and 2,500 calories are consumed on a daily basis. This means that the calories on non-working days range from 400 to 500. For those who enjoy working out every day, intermittent fasting is not recommended. On your off days, you'll have to limit your activity.

When you first begin this intermittent fasting method, you can get through low-calorie days by drinking protein shakes. Eating 'real' foods, as opposed to shakes, is better for you these days.

Weight loss is the focus of intermittent fasting. People who try it lose two to three pounds per week on average, according to reports. If you're going to try the Alternate Day Diet, it's critical that you eat full-calorie meals. If you continue to binge, you will not only be unable to see your progress, but you will also be risking serious bodily harm.

Meal Missing

If you don't have a regular schedule or aren't sure if intermittent fasting is right for you, intermittent fasting is a good way to get started. While strict fasting is necessary for the best results, there are other advantages.

After you've tried intermittent fasting, you'll be able to see the advantages for yourself. This may assist you in making future positive changes. Intermittent fasting has a wide range of possibilities. There's a good chance you'll find one that works for you. Except for a few unimportant pounds, you don't need to lose anything?

Intermittent Fasting Foods to Stay Away From

The foods listed below should be avoided or minimized to the greatest extent possible.

Non-Organic Milk: Despite its popularity as part of a well-balanced diet, non-organic milk frequently contains growth hormones and 'pusses' as a result of over-milking. Hormones that stimulate growth

Antibiotics are left behind, making the body's fight against infections more difficult. Breast cancer, prostate cancer, and colon cancer become more likely as a result.

White flour has no nutritional value once it has been processed, just like processed meats. According to Care2, women who consume white flour as part of their regular diet have a 200 percent increased risk of breast cancer.

Processed meats: While protein is necessary for a balanced diet, eating processed meats will overburden your body with chemicals. Processed meats have a lower protein content and a higher sodium content than fresh meats. They also contain preservatives, which have been linked to a variety of health issues, such as heart disease and asthma. In grocery stores, you can select from the highest-quality cuts of meat.

Non-Organic Potatoes - While the starch, carbohydrates, and vitamins found in non-organic potatoes are important in a well-balanced diet, they aren't worth the effort. They're buried and chemically treated. The potatoes are then taken to the store and kept as "fresh" as possible. These chemicals have been linked to an increased risk of learning disabilities, autism, Parkinson's disease, Alzheimer's disease, birth defects, and other cancers.

Farm-Raised Salmon - Like processed meats, farm-raised fish is the healthiest option for a balanced meal. Salmon raised in close quarters lose a lot of their natural vitamin D and can pick up trace amounts of PCB, DDT, carcinogens, and bromine. These are just a few of the reasons why processed foods should not be seen as a problem in today's society. Processed food is defined as any food that contains artificial colors, flavors, preservatives, or additives. A high carbohydrate content in a food item means it's unhealthy.

Fasting for Weight Loss: A Step-by-Step Guide

These are self-evident but crucial:
Maintain a calorie deficit: This is true for all diets, but intermittent fasting is particularly risky because it's easy to overeat and undo any gains. You'll need to eat an average of 3,500 calories per week to lose one pound per week.

During fasting, stick to the same schedule. It is critical to stick to whatever method of weight loss you choose. If you try intermittent fasting with the Paleo diet for a few days before switching to a lower-carb diet, your body will be confused.

The best way to reap the benefits of fasting is to do so on a regular basis. Only after your body has had time to adjust to the new routine will you be able to adjust. This can improve the neural pathways that lead to weight loss by increasing the amount of positive enzymes in your body.

To achieve proactive weight loss success, you must be consistent.

Avoid junk food: While intermittent fasting allows you to eat more junk food, doing so is a recipe for disaster. Although you may be able to reduce your calorie intake, it is preferable to avoid junk food and save calories by exercising.

not on foods that will stick to your ribs for an extended period of time. Consume foods rich in protein and healthy fats. For longer periods of time, you will feel more full and energetic. Each day has a limited amount of time. Make a good impression.

Maintain your self-control: Intermittent fasting only works if you fast for a maximum of twelve hours. The cycle will be reset by any caloric intact. Controlling your urges is critical if you want to see real results with this approach. You won't be able to eat as much or as little as usual if you fast for only twelve hours. Nothing you see can be eaten. It's crucial to control your appetite if you want to be successful.

Profits to be had

Intermittent fasting is an excellent way to gain muscle and shed pounds. You can free up time by getting up earlier and eating breakfast every morning. Although it may appear difficult to give up your morning breakfast, new habits can be formed that make it seem as simple as pie. The following are just a few of the many reasons to fast:

Cortisol production has decreased, lowering stress levels.

Improved Heart Health: This plan can lower blood triglycerides, LDL cholesterol, insulin resistance, and blood sugar levels. Each of these is a major risk factor for heart disease and other illnesses.

The process was only tested on animals, which is a plus for anti-aging. Fasted rats, on the other hand, lived 36 to 83 percent longer than non-fasted rats.

Insulin resistance is increased. These figures suggest that you should be better protected against type 2 diabetes and have a consistent level of energy and mood.

"Your brain hormone, BDNF, also known as brain-derived neurotropic factor (or "neurotropic") factor, can aid in the growth and maintenance of nerve cells," according to Science Daily. Fasting may help people with Parkinson's disease and Alzheimer's disease.

Inflammation is decreased: Inflammation is the root of many chronic diseases. Ketogenic diet methods have been shown to reduce swelling in private studies. Your body will be able to heal, repair, and recover faster as a result of the diet plan than it would be otherwise.

Acceleration of Fatty Acid Oxidation - Your body will burn more fat for energy, and you will lose weight quickly.
The body will begin to repair your cells by eliminating all waste. HGH (Human Growth Hormone): This hormone is found in the blood and causes levels to rise. It will aid in fat loss as well as muscle growth.

Cancer patients are in the best possible position: there is still hope for cancer patients. Fasting for a short period of time has been shown to help prevent certain diseases.

Animal studies support this.

You can see that intermittent fasting has numerous advantages, including weight loss and a variety of other unique advantages that you can enjoy while on the ketogenic diet. You will live longer and have improved biological functions if you can achieve extended fasting.

Keep in mind that your strategy will not leave you hungry. The emergency signals sent by your body are only that: signals. Once your body has adjusted to the intermittent fasting diet you've chosen, you'll see a decrease in fasting.

Note: These research projects are still in the early stages. To confirm the benefits of fasting, human testing is needed. Do you see the similarities between the two methods of fasting and ketogenic cooking?

Is It Actually Effective?

Because of hormonal changes ranging from 3.6 percent to 14 percent, short-term fasting increases your metabolic rate. Three to 24 weeks of intermittent fasting resulted in weight loss of 3.0 to 8.0 percent, according to research. In comparison to other weight-loss studies, these are significant percentages that should not be overlooked.

During the same study, many of these people lost between 4% and 7% of their waist circumference. This demonstrates how dangerous belly fat accumulations can lead to disease and other issues in the areas surrounding your organs. This can be accomplished by eating fewer calories overall and avoiding weekend binges. A healthy diet is essential.

Intermittent fasting Should Be Avoided

Intermittent fasting, like many other aspects of life, may not be right for you. If you work in these areas, you may need to lift the restrictions:

Those who have struggled with an eating disorder

When taken on an empty stomach, prescription medications can cause issues. Diabetics who take metformin may experience nausea and diarrhea. Supplementing with iron can also cause stomach upset. Aspirin can also cause stomach upset and ulcers in some people.

Type 1 or type 2 diabetics It's more likely to happen to people who have had a lot of blood sugar drops.

Those who are underweight (BMI 18.5), malnourished, or suffer from other nutrient deficiencies

For the unborn child, pregnant women will require more nutrition. Breastfeeding mothers will require additional nutrients for their children.

The growth of children under the age of 18 necessitates more nutrients.

Adequate Fluid Intake Is Very Important

When you're on a fasting program like this, you'll need to stay hydrated. Although clear liquids are appealing, they lack essential nutrients. Only apple juice, water, and broth are permitted to be consumed.

Days are moving quickly. You'll be fasting for 20 to 24 hours, so you should be able to do it.

Ice cream, skim milk, pulp juice, and strained creamy soup are also available. You could also try a whey protein supplement shake or a low-fat frozen yogurt. These foods will provide essential nutrients and fiber, as well as the necessary calorie amounts. Use low-calorie juices, ice cream, and a few cubes to make a delectable smoothie.

It is best to seek medical advice before beginning any diet or other type of dieting. You may need to stop taking medications or dietary supplements while fasting. Daily liquid diets can provide between 400 and 800 calories, according to Vanderbilt University research.

Extra Pointers

During this fasting period, it's critical to refrain from binging and fasting. This

will wreak havoc on your internal organs. This is an excessive amount of effort for your body to handle. Only people who can control their food intake and exercise moderation can use the cycle. When you aren't fasting, the experts recommend doing resistance-style weight training.

Try a light yoga or cardio session if you feel completely out of your routine on fasting days. It may be difficult for you to adhere to your fasting schedule if you are unable to exercise as much. Anxiety, fatigue, and headaches are common at first. This will go away once your body has adjusted to the new diet. Remember that each day you stick to your plan successfully is a day closer to your goal.

Success Prescriptions

Plan your menus ahead of time to ensure the best possible combination of foods. To make your complete menu plan, combine vegetables and protein. It's impossible to combine starch, sugar, fat, and gluten in a healthy way.

Combinations that Worked in the Past Beans and eggs are a classic combination. nut and seed combinations
Potatoes with eggs

Whey Protein and Berries Peanut butter with cocoa nibs Peas and potatoes are two of the most popular vegetables in the United States. Wine with nuts

Wine and cheese are a classic combination. Examples of Bad Combinations: Rice and Beans

Wine and pasta Pasta with almonds
Nuts, raisins (trail mixture)

Cream, sugar, and
Peanut butter with jelly Bread with jam.

Sour cream, potatoes, and granola (honey nut)

Intermittent fasting and the ketogenic methods used to achieve it will become more familiar to you as time goes on. Allow for some time to pass.
Fasting Rules That Are Simple to Follow

Maintain Control: Regardless of which intermittent fasting method you use, you must ask yourself if you are capable of adhering to the necessary diet plans in order to maintain a healthy food intake. If you want to reach a 500-calorie daily deficit, you must curb your appetite. You won't have much of a window to eat your next meal if you skip a meal.

Keep a Calorie Tally: If you don't keep track of your calories, you might find yourself overeating at meals. You must burn more calories than you consume each week to lose one pound.

Continue to stick to the pre-determined course of action. A regular fasting schedule must be established. If you change plans, your body will adjust to the new method. When you change from a 5:2 to a 16:8 diet, your body will stop losing weight until it adjusts to the new plan. You will be wasting time if you switch. Consistency is crucial for a successful fasting plan.

Chapter 3: Keto Breakfast Specialties

1. Included is a pdf file

2. In your summary section, you will find the pdf version. It allows you to print the recipes as well as the book's 7-Day Meal Plan and Shopping List.

3. Wrap made with bacon, spinach, avocado, and an egg

4.

5. 2 Servings (approx.)

6. 672 calories, 4 grams of net carbohydrates, 33 grams of total protein, and 57 grams of total fats Ingredients Needed:

7. Large eggs - 2 Bacon - 6 slices

8. whipped cream (heavy) 2 tablespoons (tbsp.)

9. 1 tbsp butter (or as many as necessary)

10.

11.   Fresh spinach or a favorite choice - 1 cup Sliced avocado -.

12.

13.   5 out of 1\sFreshly cracked black pepper and Pink Himalayan salt to your liking

14.   Preparation Tips:

15.

16.   To cook the bacon, heat the stovetop on medium heat for approximately 8 minutes. Use a towel to drain the grease off the bacon.

17.

18.   Mix the cream, eggs and salt together. Pour half of the mixture into the greased skillet. Cook until set (1 min) (1 min.) Flip. If necessary, add more butter. Cook the second egg for 1 minute more per side. Place the egg on a towel.

19.

20.   Place the avocado slices and bacon spinach on a plate. Serve immediately. Biscuits & Gravy Included is a pdf file

21.   In your summary section, you will find the pdf version. It allows you to print the recipes as well as the book's 7-Day Meal Plan and Shopping List.

22.   Wrap made with bacon, spinach, avocado, and an egg

23.

24.   2 Servings (approx.)

25. 672 calories, 4 grams of net carbohydrates, 33 grams of total protein, and 57 grams of total fats Ingredients Needed:

26. Large eggs - 2 Bacon - 6 slices

27. whipped cream (heavy) 2 tablespoons (tbsp.)

28. 1 tbsp butter (or as many as necessary)

29.

30. Fresh spinach or a favorite choice - 1 cup Sliced avocado -.

31.

32. 5 out of 1\sFreshly cracked black pepper and Pink Himalayan salt to your liking

33. Preparation Tips:

34.

35. To cook the bacon, heat the stovetop on medium heat for approximately 8 minutes. Use a towel to drain the grease off the bacon.

36.

37. Mix the cream, eggs and salt together. Pour half of the mixture into the greased skillet. Cook until set (1 min) (1 min.) Flip. If necessary, add more butter. Cook the second egg for 1 minute more per side. Place the egg on a towel.

38.

39. Place the avocado slices and bacon spinach on a plate. Serve immediately. Biscuits & Gravy

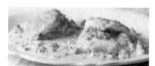

Total Macros: 425 Calories| 2 g Net Carbs | 22 g Total Protein | 36 g Total Fats Ingredients Needed:

Salt - .25 tsp.\sAlmond flour - 0.25 cup Baking powder-.5 teaspoon. Large egg whites - 1

Crumbled breakfast sausage 6 oz. Chicken broth - .25 cup Cream cheese - .25 cup

1. How to prepare:

2. Heat the oven to 400oF. Bake in a pan with parchment paper.

3. Mix the almond flour, salt, and baking powder together.

4. Whisk the egg whites in another dish until you get stiff peaks.

5. Cut the butter into small pieces. Use the butter to make a crumbly mixture. Blend the dry ingredients into the egg whites.

6. Divide the batter into two parts and place them on a parchmentlined pan. Bake for between 11 and 15 minutes.

7. Warm the sausage on medium heat. Once the sausage is browned, add the cream cheese and chicken broth. Let it simmer for a few minutes, then season with salt and pepper.

8. Serve the hot biscuits with deliciousgravy.

9. The prep time for this recipe is only 15 minutes and the cooking time is only 25 minutes. This is a great way to enjoy a delicious meal in a short time! Blueberry Ricotta Pancakes

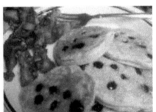

1. There are 5 servings in this recipe.

2. 311 calories | 6 grams of net carbs | 15 grams of total protein | 23 grams of total fats

3.

4. Large eggs - 3 Unsweetened vanilla almond milk -.25 cup Golden flaxseed meal -.5 cup Salt -.25 tsp

5.

6. 1 teaspoon baking powder 1 cup almond flour +.5 teaspoon stevia powder .5 teaspoon vanilla extract .25 cup blueberries

7. Your preferred keto-friendly syrup - If you want to add carbs, do so as follows:

8.

9. To combine the eggs, milk, and ricotta, use an electric mixer.

10. Combine the flaxseed meal, salt, flour, baking powder, and stevia in a separate dish.

11. Slowly pour the dry ingredients into the blender to make the batter. Use two to three blueberries per pancake.

12.

13. In a skillet, melt the butter on the medium heat setting. After the butter has melted, scoop

two tablespoons of batter into a skillet.

14.

15.   Serve immediately or set aside to cool.

16.   If you're short on time, the syrup can be frozen and used later. If you know your schedule is packed, you can use a cup with a lid. 7. Toss some bacon into your favorite dish and add some carbs. Coffee that is bulletproof

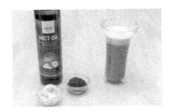

2. 320 calories | 0 g net carbs | 1 g total protein | 51 g total fats The following are the necessary ingredients for this recipe:

3. 2 teaspoons MCT oil powder 2 tablespoons ghee/butter

4. 1.5 cups of coffee, hot

5.

6. Preparation Tips:

7. In a blender, mix the hot coffee.

8. Combine the butter and the powder in a large mixing bowl. Until smooth, blend.

9. Make sure you have a big mug for this.

10.   Eggs à la crème

11.

12.   1 serving: 341 calories, 3 grams of net carbs, 15 grams of total protein, and 31 grams of total fats

13.

14.   – 1 tbsp. butter 2 eggs 2 tablespoons soft cream cheese with chives

15.

16.   Preparation Tips:

17.   In a skillet, melt the butter. Combine the cream cheese and eggs in a mixing bowl. 2. Combine all of the ingredients in a pan and whisk until they're the consistency you want. 'Fatty' Omelet with Full Herbing

18.

19.   1 serving (about a quarter of a cup of water)

20.   719 calories, 3.3 grams of net carbohydrates, 30 grams of total protein, and 63 grams of total fats The following are the necessary ingredients for this recipe:

21.   2 large eggs -.5 cup grated Parmesan cheese - 1 tbsp. basil 2 tablespoons ghee

22.   .5 tbsp oregano (freshly chopped)

23.

24.   1 tblsp. salt 1 slice crisp bacon 1 tblsp. avocado Preparation Tips:

25.

26. Parmesan cheese, grated In a large mixing bowl, combine the eggs and herbs. Combine the oregano, basil, and parmesan cheeses in a large mixing bowl.

27. Warm a skillet over medium-high heat. Reduce the heat to medium-low and stir in the cranberries.

28.

29. egg.

30. Heat the aspatula for 30 seconds to bring the egg to the middle of the pan. When the egg is solid enough to flip, do so. Cook for 30 seconds at a minimum. 4. Garnish with sliced avocado and crisp bacon. Soups and Salads for Lunch (Chapter 4)

31. Have a salad or a bowl soup if you don't feel like eating a complete meal.

32.

33. 4 servings of Creamy Chicken Soup

34. 307 calories, 2 grams of net carbohydrates, 18 grams of total protein, and 25 grams of total fat The following are the necessary ingredients for this recipe:

35. − 2 tblsp. butter

36. 1 to 2 cups shredded large chicken breast 4 ounces of cubed cheese

37.

38. 2 tablespoons garlic seasoning; 14.5 ounces chicken broth season with salt according your preference

39. Use 1.25 cup heavy cream Preparation Tips:

40.

41. In a skillet over medium heat, melt the butter.

42. Combine the shredded chicken and cream cheese in a large mixing bowl. In a large mixing bowl, combine the cream cheese and spices.

43. Add the heavy whipping cream and broth after the mixture has melted. 4. Reduce the heat to low and cook for three to four minutes after the water has boiled. As desired, season. Instant Pot No-Beans Beef Chili

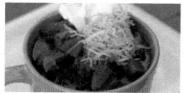

8 Servings (about)

326 calories, 8 grams of net carbohydrates, 23 grams of total protein, and 17 grams of total fats The following are the necessary ingredients for this recipe:

1 medium chopped onion or dried onion flakes (optional).

2 lbs. 5 cup beef

2 cans (15 oz.) of tomato sauce 1 tsp. Tabasco

a 6 oz. jar of tomato paste

1 tblsp. of garlic powder 2 chili powders – 5 tbsp. or minced cloves

cumin powder, 1 tbsp 1 teaspoon oregano, dried 2 teaspoons sea salt, finely ground

Chicken or beef broth may be used to thin the sauce.

1. Preparation Tips:
2.
3. Cut the onion into small pieces. Use the Instant Pot's sauté setting to brown the meat. Add the Tabasco sauce and onion flakes and stir to combine. Salt, chili powder, cumin, and Tabasco sauce should all be added at this point. Make a thorough mixture. Completely combine all ingredients.
4.
5. Do not whisk the tomato paste and sauce together.
6. Allow 10 minutes for the manual high pressure setting to run.
7. Simply let the pressure out naturally for 10 minutes before suddenly letting it out.
8. Serve with a stir.
9.
10.   Caprese Salad for Lunch 4 Servings (about)
11.   191 calories, 4.6 grams of net carbohydrates, 7.7 grams of total protein, and 63.5 grams of total fats The following are the necessary ingredients for this recipe:
12.   a third of a cup of grape tomatoes 4 garlic cloves, peeled – 2 tablespoons avocado oil
13.   19 pearl-size mozzarella balls
14.
15.   4 CUP BABY SPROUTING SPROUTING SPROUTING SPROUT .25 CUP FRESH BASIL
16.   1 tbsp. cheese (reserved) a tblsp. of pesto Preparation tips:
17.
18.   Use aluminum foil to protect a baking sheet.
19.   Preheat oven to 400 degrees Fahrenheit (200 degrees Celsius).
20.   Drizzle the olive oil over the tomatoes and garlic cloves on a baking sheet. Cook for 20-30 minutes, or until gently browned on top.
21.   One tablespoon of the juice from the mozzarella should be set aside. Combine the pesto and the brine in a bowl and stir to combine.
22.   In a large mixing basin, toss the spinach. In a separate bowl, combine the tomatoes and roasted garlic. Combine the pesto sauce and the other ingredients in a large mixing bowl.
23.   Fresh basil leaves and mozzarella balls may be added to the meal as a garnish.
24.   Cobb Salad is a kind of salad that is often served

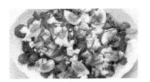

1. 2 Servings (about.)

2. 600 calories, 3 grams of net carbohydrates, 43 grams of total protein, and 48 grams of total fat

3.

4. The following are the necessary ingredients for this recipe:

5.

6. 1 hard-boiled egg – 1 cup spinach – 2 campari tomatoes –.5 off 1 chicken breasts – 2 oz. 1 tbsp. avocado, 1.25 avocado, 1.25 avocado, avocado, avocado, avocado, avocado, avocado, avocado, avocado, avocado, avocado, avocado, avocado, avocado,

7.

8. 0.5 teaspoon white vinegar Preparation tips:

9.

10.   1. Prepare the chicken and bacon. Cut the chicken into slices. 2. Cut all of the ingredients into tiny pieces. Combine the ingredients with the oil and vinegar in a mixing bowl. Serve after giving them a little toss. salad made with kale

11.

12.   4 Servings (200 g) Carbohydrates (net)

13.   1 tbsp olive oil,.5 teaspoon salt

14.

15.   1 bunch kale - 1 tablespoon lemon juice - 1 tablespoon Parmesan cheese

16.

17.   Cut the kale into 1/4-inch strips after removing the ribs.

18.   Toss for 3 minutes after combining the oil and salt.

19.   Combine the cheese, kale, and salt in a mixing bowl. Serve. Salad Keto in King-Size

20.

21.   2 Servings (about.)

22.   581 calories, 9 grams of net carbohydrates, 38 grams of total protein, and 43 grams of total fats The following are the necessary ingredients for this recipe:

23. 2 sliced avocado - 2 boneless chicken breasts - 6 finely sliced bacon slices - 1

24.

25. 4 cups mixed leafy greens Dressing for keto ranch a fourth of a teaspoon Preparation tips:

26.

27. Preheat oven to 400 degrees Fahrenheit (200 degrees Celsius).

28. Melt the ghee in a large pan, then add the skin-side-down chicken. Cook for 30 seconds after flipping the chicken.

29. Preheat the oven to 350 degrees Fahrenheit and place the skillet inside. Preheat the oven to 350 degrees Fahrenheit and bake for 10 to 15 minutes. Internal temperature should be attained at 165 degrees Fahrenheit.

30. Prepare a baking dish with parchment paper. 10 minutes on a baking tray, bake the bacon slices. This recipe is also suitable.

31. Cut the chicken and avocado in half. Begin by layering the greens, avocado, and chicken on top of the salad.

32.

33. With a couple teaspoons of dressing on top, it's a delicious meal.

34.

35. Salad of Lobster

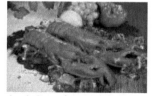

1. 4 Servings (about)

2. 307 calories, 2 grams of net carbs, 18 grams of total protein, and 25 grams of total fats are the total macronutrients. The following are the necessary ingredients for this recipe:

3. 1 pound cooked lobster flesh, melted butter –.25 cup .25 cup of mayonnaise

4.

5. pepper, black

6.

7. 1 tablespoon (125 tsp) Cut the lobster into little pieces to make it easier to cook.

8. In a large mixing basin, put the meat. Combine the mayonnaise, salt, and pepper in a large mixing bowl.

9.

10.   Chill for at least 10 minutes with the dish covered.

11.

12.   Salad with Tuna

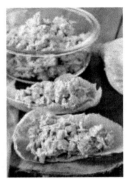

2 Servings (about.)

465 calories, 6 grams of net carbs, 68.5 grams of total protein, and 18.1 grams of total fats The following are the necessary ingredients for this recipe:

2 cans (15 oz each) tuna in oil 1 tablespoon olive oil

2 tbsp lemon juice (freshly squeezed) a mouthful

2 boiled eggs, finely chopped Cucumbers, sliced – 1/5

1 medium or 2 bigger red onions, thinly sliced

2 tbsp. mayonnaise, 2 tbsp. dijon mustard

Preparation Tips:

Tuna should be drained. Mix the oil, lemon juice, and mayonnaise together in a container. Combine all remaining ingredients in a mixing bowl. Refrigerate for a while.

When you're ready to dine, pour the dressing over the salad. Combine the salad ingredients by tossing it together. Club Salad for Vegetarians

3 servings (about).

330 calories, 5 grams of net carbohydrates, 17 grams of total protein, and 26 grams of total fats

The following are the necessary ingredients for this recipe: – 2 tbsp. mayonnaise 2 teaspoon garlic powder 1 teaspoon of dried parsley a half teaspoon of onion powder 1 teaspoon of milk 1 tablespoon dijon mustard

3 large hard-boiled eggs– 4 oz.

3 cups torn Romaine lettuce,.5 cup cherry tomatoes, 1 cup diced cucumber Preparation Tips:

Hard-boiled eggs should be sliced in half, and the cheese should be cut in half. Cut the tomatoes in half and slice the cucumbers. Set the containers to the side for the time being.

Combine the dried herbs, mayonnaise, and sour cream in a large mixing bowl.

Add 1 tbsp milk to the mix. Add another tablespoon if it becomes too dry.

Cheese, veggies, and eggs are layered in the salad. In the center, pour a spoonful of mustard.

Drizzle some dressing over the top.

Toss everything together and eat it up!

Notes: Nutritional numbers are based on 2 tbsp.

dressing.

Appetizers

Asparagus & Garlic

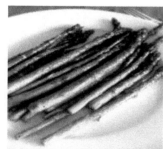Yields: 4 Servings

1. Carbohydrates (net): 2 g

2.

3. 1 tablespoon minced garlic 1 bunch of raw asparagus 2 tbsp. margarine

4.

5. Preparation Tips:

6.

7. After rinsing, separate the asparagus stems. For 2-3 minutes, boil the asparagus. Drain the water and place in a dish of ice water to chill.

1. Melt the butter and garlic in a large pan. In a skillet with butter and garlic, cook the asparagus until it is golden brown. Servings: 4 Macros: Buffalo Cauliflower Bites 130 calories | 3 g Net Carbs | 12 g Fat | 2 g Protein Cauliflower florets (four cups) are required. – to taste – cracked black pepper .25 teaspoons salt .25 teaspoon cayenne

2.

3. 4 teaspoons salted butter 1 clove minced garlic and.25 cup hot sauce .25 tsp paprika

4. Blue cheese dressing is an optional ingredient.

5.

6. Preheat oven to 375 degrees Fahrenheit.

7.

8. In a baking pan lined with parchment, place the florets.

9. Combine the spicy sauce, cayenne, garlic, salt, paprika, and butter in a mixing bowl. Combine the remaining ingredients in a blender and blend until smooth.

10.   After baking the florets for 25 minutes, pour the sauce over them. 5. Serve a cup of blue cheese dressing on the side as a dipping sauce. Mac and Cheese with Cauliflower

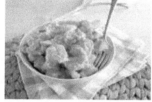

4 Servings (about)

294 calories, 7 grams of net carbohydrates, 11 grams of total protein, and 23 grams of total fats The following are the necessary ingredients for this recipe:

– 3 tblsp. butter

1 cup cheddar cheese Cauliflower – 1 head

To experience: salt with black pepper

Almond milk (unsweetened) –

Use a quarter of a gallon of heavy cream

Cup 25 Preparation Tips:

After that, shred the cheese and cut the cauliflower into little florets.

It's a good idea to pre-set the oven temperature to 450 degrees Fahrenheit.

Use aluminum foil or parchment paper to cover a baking pan.

2 tablespoons butter, melted Toss the florets with the butter. Using salt and pepper, give

the cauliflower a thorough shake. For 10-15 minutes, roast the cauliflower.

In a microwave or double boiler, melt the remaining butter, milk, and heavy cream. 6. Finally, pour the cheese in the bowl. Greek Salad with Chopped Onions

2 Servings (about.)

202 calories, 2 grams of net carbs, 4 grams of total protein, and 19 grams of total fats The following are the necessary ingredients for this recipe:

Halved grape tomatoes - .5 cup Chopped romaine – 2 cups

Kalamata Black Olives - 1.25 Cup Crumbled Feta Cheese - 1.25 Cup Olive Oil - 1 Tbsp.

Vinaigrette dressing - 2 tbsp.

To your taste, black pepper and pink salt

How to Prepare:

1. As a base, prepare the salad using the romaine. You can make it as you like and drizzle some oil or vinegar on top.

2. Enjoy with two salads.Chapter 5: Dinnertime Favorites

You can choose from beef, pork, or poultry for your meal preparation.

Beef2 cups chopped romaine lettuce, halved grape tomatoes

1.25 cup kalamata black olives, 1.25 cup crumbled feta cheese, 1.25 cup olive oil, 1 tablespoon olive oil 2 tbsp vinaigrette

Black pepper and pink salt, according to your preferences.

Make the salad using romaine as a basis. You may prepare it whatever you like and top it with olive oil or vinegar.

Toss two salads together and serve.

Dinnertime Classics (Chapter 5)

Meal preparation options include beef, pork, and chicken.

Cheeseburger with Beef and Bacon

Bacon Cheeseburger

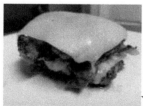
Yields 12 servings - 2 burgers per person

489 calories, 0.8 grams of net carbs, 27 grams of total protein, and 41 grams of total fats The following are the necessary ingredients for this recipe:

3 lb. lean ground beef

16 oz. packet of low-sodium bacon 2 eggs - 0.5 medium chopped onion - 8 oz. Preparation Tips:

desired. Make a double-decker if you have the extra carbs. It tastes fantastic! Instant Pot Barbecue Beef

9 Servings (approximately)

153 calories, 2 grams of net carbohydrates, 24 grams of total protein, and 4.5 grams of total fats

The following are the necessary ingredients for this recipe:

3 lb. roast eye round/bottom round to taste black pepper 2.5 tsp. Kosher salt 1 cup water

0.5 out of 1 onion, medium

Lime – 1 garlic clove, juiced – 5 chipotles in adobo sauce – taste and adjust as needed. 1 tbsp oregano 1 tablespoon ground cumin

3 ground cloves – 0.5 teaspoon Oil – 1 tsp. Bay leaves – 1 tsp

Preparation Tips:

To program your Instant Pot, use the saute function.

3 inch pieces of beef should be sliced Salt and pepper to taste.

A blender should be used to combine the water, spices, chilies, limejuice, onion, and garlic. Cook for five minutes with the meat in the pan with the oil. Add the bay leaf and the sauce (from your blender).

With the top removed, cook the mixture for 65 minutes in saute mode. You can continue cooking once it can easily be shredded with two forks. Add more water if needed to keep it moist.

Place the mixture on a platter and shred it after it has finished cooking. The bay leaves can be discarded, but the juices can be saved for another time.

1.5 cup of the reserved juices, along with 1/2 teaspoon cumin and salt, should be consumed. Serve once it's warmed through and all of the flavors have melded.

Slow-cooker Chuck Steak

8 Servings (about)

667 calories, 2.9 grams of net carbohydrates, 79 grams of total protein, and 33 grams of total fats

The following are the necessary ingredients for this recipe:

4.4 lb. of chuck steak a stalk of celery 2 cups beef stock – 4 carrots – 3 garlic cloves

red wine, one glass

To taste, add salt and pepper.

Preparation Tips:

Fill the cooker halfway with water. Cook on high for 4 hours with the roast in the cooker. Place the vegetables around the roast in small pieces.

Combine the broth and wine with all of the spices.

Cook on high for another four hours.

Serve the steak with the vegetables, which should be cut into eight portions.

Stroganoff of Hamburger

1 serving (about a quarter of a cup of water)

447 calories, 6 grams of net carbohydrates, 39 grams of total protein, and 28 grams of total fat The following are the necessary ingredients for this recipe:

1 pound, 8 ounces lean ground beef 2 tablespoons butter, minced garlic cloves 1 1/4 cup sour cream

1 tsp. lemon juice or a glass of dry white wine 1 teaspoon of parsley, dry

.25 tsp paprika

1 tbsp. parsley, freshly chopped Preparation tips:

Sauté the garlic and onions in 1 tablespoon butter in a large skillet. Butter.

In a separate pan, brown the beef. If desired, season to taste with salt and pepper. Cook until the beef is tender.

In the same pan, add the butter, mushrooms, and wine/water. Cook until the mushrooms are softened and the liquid is reduced by half.

Remove from heat and stir in the paprika or sour cream.

Over low heat, incorporate the meat and lemon zest. Add more spices to the mix.

if desired, flavoring

Poultry

Chicken Breast with Garlic & Parsley

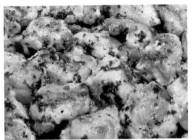

1. 4 Servings (about)

2. 150 calories, 4.1 grams of net carbohydrates, 25 grams of total protein, and 3.1 grams of total fats The following are the necessary ingredients for this recipe:

3. 2 tbsp parsley, 2 tbsp basil, 2 tbsp parsley, 2 tbsp basil, 2 tbsp parsley, 2 tbsp parsley, 2

4. .5 teaspoons salt

5. 4 minced garlic cloves for chicken breast halves, boneless and skinless garlic

6.

7. .5 teaspoon of crushed red pepper flakes Tomatoes, sliced (two)

8. A 9x13-inch baking dish is also necessary. Preparation tips:

9.

10.   Preheat oven to 350 degrees Fahrenheit (180 degrees Celsius).

11.   Use cooking spray to coat the casserole dish. On the plate, scatter half of the basil and half of the parsley.

12.   Add the garlic and chicken to the pan.

13.   Combine the basil, parsley, and red pepper with the basil and salt in a large mixing bowl.

14.   On top of the chicken, spread the tomato slices.

15.

16.   With a cover on, bake for 25 minutes.

17.   Before serving, bake for another 15 minutes on top.

18.   Nuggets of Chicken

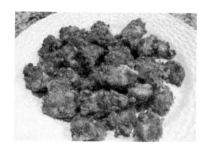

1. 6 Servings (approximately)

2. 243 calories, 2 grams of net carbohydrates, 18 grams of total protein, and 17 grams of total fats
The following are the necessary ingredients for this recipe:

4.

5. Preparation Tips:

6.

7. Preheat oven to 350 degrees Fahrenheit (180 degrees Celsius).

8. Using a cooking oil or spray, lightly coat a baking sheet. You could also use parchment paper to layer it on top.

9. To shred the chicken, use a stand mixer or a food processor. Depending on your preferences, you can use a mix of white and darker meat.

10. Combine all of the remaining ingredients in a large mixing bowl and thoroughly combine them. 5. Fill a baking pan halfway with the nugget mixture. Bake for 12-14 minutes, or until the nugget mixture is golden brown. 12-14 minutes in the oven Creamy Chicken & Greens

11.

12. 4 Servings (about)

13. 446 calories, 2.6 grams of net carbs, 18.4 grams of total protein, and 38 grams of total fat
The following are the necessary ingredients for this recipe:

14. – 2 tbsp. coconut oil

15. 1 pound of boneless chicken thighs with skins To taste, season with salt and pepper. 2 tablespoons melted butter

16.

17. 1 cup chicken stock 2 tablespoons coconut flour 2 cups dark leafy greens, 1 cup cream, 1 teaspoon Italian herbs Preparation tips:

18.

19. In a large skillet over high heat, heat the oil. Bring to a boil. The chicken should be

seasoned with salt and pepper. Cook until the chicken is golden brown on medium heat.

20.

21. Toss in the butter and stir the sauce together. Combine the flour and water in a blender until a thick paste is formed. Whisk in the cream, one tablespoon at a time, until smooth. After it's boiled, add the herbs.

22.

23. Transfer the chicken to the counter after adding the stock. In a saucepan, combine all of the ingredients for the cream sauce.

24.

25. Combine the greens and sauce in a bowl.

26.

27. On the greens, place the thighs. Serve hot. Pork

Carnitas– Crockpot

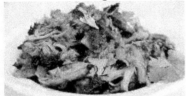

1. 2 Servings (about.)

2. 446 calories, 4 grams of net carbs, 45 grams of total protein, and 26 grams of total fats The following are the necessary ingredients for this recipe:

3.

4. 1 pound boneless pork butt roast.5 teaspoon chili powder 1 tbsp. of olive oil

5. 1 lime juice + 1 small diced onion + 1 minced garlic clove + 1 lime juice + 1 lime juice + 1 lime juice + 1 lime juice + 1 lime juice + 1 lime juice + 1 lime juice + 1 lime juice + 1 lime juice + 2

6. To experience: black pepper, pink salt

7. Preparation Tips:

8.

9. Use the low temperature setting in the crockpot to warm it.

10. Combine the chili powder and the olive oil in a mixing bowl. Rub the pork all over and place it in the oven, fat side up.

11. Combine the vegetables, salt, lime juice, and pepper in a mixing bowl.

12. Allow to simmer for 8 hours on low heat, covered.

13. Shred the meat on a cutting board with two forks once it's done cooking.

14. Take a lettuce leaf and eat it, but don't forget to include some carbs. 7. The cooking time is 8 hours and the total prep time is only 10 minutes. Cauli Rice Luau Pork Luau

15.

16. 9 Servings (approximately)

17. 182 calories, 1.1 grams of net carbs, 14 grams of total protein, and 13 grams of total fats The following are the necessary ingredients for this recipe:

18. 4 slices of hickory-smoked bacon 3 lb. roast shoulder/pork 1-2 tablespoons Hawaiian black lava salt

19.

20. 4-6 cloves minced garlic

21. Optional: hickory liquid smoking a couple of tablespoons Rice needs the following ingredients: 2 tbsp chicken broth (homemade/organic) 3 cups of cauliflower 0.125 teaspoon of salt

22. 0.25 teaspoon garlic powder Preparation tips:

23.

24. High heat is an option for the slow cooker. In the bottom of the pan, layer the garlic cloves and bacon slices.

25. Place the black lava salt in a small container. In a small container, pour the black lava salt. Cover the smoker with liquid smoke for 2 hours on high or 4–6 hours on low (low). The bone-in process could take up to ten hours.

26. Remove the bones from the pork and shred it to make sure it's fully cooked. Cook for another 30 minutes at a low temperature.

27. You can now start preparing the rice. Rice can be steamed or microwaved for 5 minutes. Add the chicken broth, sea salt, garlic, or ginger to the slightly cooled product in the food processor. After that, process it until it resembles rice.

28. Side by side, serve the pork.

29. 4 servings of stuffed pork chops

30.

31. 778 calories, 1 gram of net carbs, 102 grams of total protein, and 38 grams of total fats The following are the necessary ingredients for this recipe:

32.

33. 3 slices sliced bacon 4 Feta cheese – 3 oz. thick cut pork chops a 3 oz. block of bleu cheese

34.

35. a 2 oz. block of cream cheese .33 cup of green onion

36. To taste, season with salt and black pepper.

37. 1 tblsp. of garlic powder Preparation tips:

38.

39. Preheat oven to 350 degrees Fahrenheit (180 degrees Celsius). The baking dish should be lightly greased.

40. Remove the bacon from the pan and set aside the fat.

41. Toss the feta and bleu cheese together. Add the onions and bacon to the mix. The cream cheese should be added after that.

42. On the non-fat side, divide the pork and top with the cheese mixture. Secure with a toothpick. Garlic powder, salt, and pepper should be sprinkled over the top.

43. In a skillet with bacon grease, sear each side for 1.5 minutes. 6. In a baking pan, place the chops. 55 minutes on the stove Allow for a three-minute resting period after removing the chops from the pan. Serve alongside a side dish of your choosing. Appetizer and Snack Options (Chapter 6)

44. Pizza with Barbequed Chicken 4 Servings (about)

45. 282 calories, 6.5 grams of net carbohydrates, 24 grams of total protein, and 16 grams of total fats The following are the necessary ingredients for this recipe:

46. 3 oz. parmesan Psyllium Husk Powder (three tablespoons) 1-2 pinches of salt & pepper

47.

48. – 6 large eggs – 1.5 teaspoon Italian seasoning 6 oz. shreddable chicken 4 tbsp. BBQ sauce

49.

50. 4 oz. cheddar 4 tbsp. of tomato sauce 1 tbsp of mayonnaise

51.

52. Preparation Tips:

53.

54. Preheat the oven to 425 degrees Fahrenheit (200 degrees Celsius).

55. Cheese should be sliced thinly. Combine the parmesan cheese, psyllium powder, and eggs in a mixing bowl with salt, pepper, and Italian seasoning. Place the dough on parchment paper to keep it from sticking to the baking pan once it has risen to a thick consistency.

56. Cook for 10 minutes on the top rack. Toss in the remaining ingredients and flip the crust over. Serve after three minutes of broiling the crust on high.

57. The pizza takes a total of 20 minutes to prepare.

58. No-Cook Cucumber Bites and Chicken-Pecan Salad

59. 2 Servings (about.)

60. 323 calories, 3 grams of net carbohydrates, 23 grams of total protein, and 24 grams of total fat

61.

62. The following are the necessary ingredients for this recipe: 2 tbsp of mayonnaise 1 cup precooked chicken breasts 1 cup diced celery 1 cup chopped pecans Preparation tips:

63.

64. Cucumber slices should be 1/4 inch thick. Celery and chicken should be chopped. Remove the pecans from their shells and chop them into small pieces. Toss the chicken, pecans, and mayonnaise together in a mixing bowl. To taste, season with salt and pepper.

65.

66. Toss the cucumber slices in a pinch of salt. A portion of the chicken salad should be layered on top of them. Serve. Bites from Pizza

67. 4 Servings (about)

68. 94 calories, 2.8 grams of net carbohydrates, 5 grams of total protein, and 7 grams of total fats

69.

70. The following are the necessary ingredients for this recipe:

71. 4 slices salami;.25 cup marinara sauce;.25 cup shredded mozzarella Preparation Tips:

72.

73. 1. Preheat the broiler in the oven to high. On a baking sheet, place the salamion. On top, put the cheese and the sauce. 2. Preheat the oven to 350°F and bake for 5 minutes. Allow them to drain the grease from the atowels for a short period of time.

74.

75. 1 to 2 minutes approximatively Serve. No-Cook Smoked Salmon and Cream Cheese Roll-Ups

76.

77. 2 Servings (about.)

78. 268 calories, 3 grams of net carbohydrates, 14 grams of total protein, and 22 grams of total fats

79.

80. The following are the necessary ingredients for this recipe: 2 tbsp. scallions, chopped (green and white parts) 1 teaspoon dijon mustard 1 teaspoon freshly grated lemon zest

81. Temp in the room a 4 oz. block of cream cheese 12 pieces of 4 oz. cold-smoked salmon

82. Depending on your preference, salt and freshly ground black pepper Preparation tips:

83.

84.   A food processor or blender can be used to combine the cream cheese, lemon zest, scallions, mustard, and milk. To taste, season with salt and pepper. Until smooth, blend.

85.   On both sides of the salmon, apply the cheese mixture. Arrange on a platter, seam side down.

86.   Place in a plastic bag and cover with plastic until you are ready to eat. They will keep

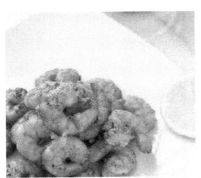

forapproximately 3 days.Zesty Shrimp
2 Servings (about.)
335 calories, 2.5 grams of
net carbohydrates, 22.5
grams of total protein, and
27 grams of total fats The
following are the necessary
ingredients for this recipe:
.25 cup extra virgin olive
oil.5 pound large shrimp
3 lemon wedges, garlic
cloves - 1 tsp. cayenne
pepper

Preparation Tips:

Toss the olive oil, garlic,
salt, and cayenne pepper
together over medium heat.
Cook each side of the
shrimp for 2-3 minutes.

Drizzle lemon juice over the shrimp and serve.

As a dipping sauce, you may use the leftover garlic oil.

BONUS 7-DAY MEAL PLAN AND SHOPPING LIST

The best approach to meal plan is with a grocery list. This is a week-to-week planning list. It may take a few weeks to stock up on all of the ketogenic diet's essentials. If you're already familiar with the ketogenic diet, you're likely to have everything you need to cook nutritious meals from this collection of recipes.

You'll need freezer bags to make storing leftovers and planning meals simpler. You may use a quality marker to date the packets to guarantee that none of the dieting supplies go to waste. You'll need the following items. These recipes may be categorized in the same way that your meal plan has been.

DAIRY DAIRY DAIRY
DAIRY DAIRY DAIRY
DAIRY DAIRY

Cream cheese -.25 cup
Ricotta -.75 cup Large eggs
- 12

Chives in a soft cream
cheese 2 tablespoons (tbsp.)
Parmesan cheese (grated) -
2 tablespoons heavy
whipping cream

6 tablespoons ghee or butter
7 SLICES BAKED
BACON
Sausage, crumbled 1 pound
of vegetables - 6 oz. ground
pork

1 cup fresh spinach or other
greens 1 tblsp. fresh basil 2
tbsp. of fresh sage
.5 teaspoon fresh oregano
FRUITS 1 blueberry plus a
little avocado Cup size: 25
CONDIMENTS
Almond milk with a hint of
vanilla.
Cup size: 25

Broth of chicken

2 tablespoons avocado oil
Coconut oil is a kind of
vegetable oil that comes
from the coconut palm 1
tbsp. olive oil
.5 tsp black pepper (freshly
cracked)

1 tsp. pink Himalayan salt /
1 pinch kosher salt

2 teaspoons finely ground
salt 1.25 tablespoons salt
2.75 cups of almond flour
2.5 tablespoons baking
powder Lavender buds fit
for a chef. 1.125 teaspoon
cayenne 1.25 tblsp. garlic
powder Or 2 golden
flaxseed meal –.5 cup
minced cloves Liquid 4
drops of stevia .5 tsp. Stevia
2 tbsp. granular sugar-free
swerve 1 tblsp. maple syrup
extract
.5 teaspoon of vanilla
extract

MCT oil powder (1 tbsp)
1.5 cups of coffee, hot

Select your preferred keto-
friendly syrup and, if
required, add the

carbohydrates. – 5 tbsp. chili powder - 2 tbsp. cumin powder

1 teaspoon oregano, dried

Lunchtime Soups and Salads (Chapter 4)

DAIRY

3 tablespoons butter, 4 tablespoons butter butter that has been salted 5 large hard-boiled eggs, 1 tablespoon of milk

5 cup of heavy cream a 4 oz. block of cream cheese 1 cup (plus) cheddar cheese 4 oz. cheddar Feta cheese,.25 cup Mozzarella balls, 19 pearl-size (+) Feta cheese,.25 cup Feta cheese,.25 cup Feta cheese,.25 cup Feta 1 tblsp. cheese brine

.33 cup grated parmesan 2 tblsp. soured cream Almond milk, unsweetened (.25 cup)

MEATS 6 boneless chicken

breasts + 3 (+) thinly chopped bacon pieces 2 lbs. of shredded beef

Anchovies, finely minced - 2 cans (15 oz. each) of tuna in oil

VEGGIES Cauliflower - 2 head (+) Cauliflower florets - 4 cups Fresh basil leaves – .25 cup Broccoli – 1 lb.

1 cauliflower romanesco (small) – divided 1 Diced cucumber 1 cup (+) Sliced cucumber (small bunch cilantro) 4 cups mixed leafy greens (1.5 cup) 5 cups of Romaine lettuce
1 medium yellow onion 3 huge red onions

3.5 cups of grape tomatoes
Five cloves of garlic 2 bunches kale
4 CUP BABY
SPROUTING
SPROUTING
SPROUTING SPROUT

1 FRUIT 1 FRUIT 1 FRUITS 1 FRUITS 1 FRUIT 1 FRUIT 1 FRUIT

1 FRU

1 tbsp. lemon juice, freshly squeezed Alternatively, to eat 3 tablespoons of seedless oranges
CONDIMENTS
1 tablespoon salted, unwashed capers .25 cup Kalamata olives 2 tbsp. garlic salt .25 teaspoon cayenne

- 10 tbsp. chili powder
2.5 teaspoon garlic powder
Cumin powder – 4 tbsp., or minced cloves – 5

2 teaspoons oregano, dried a half teaspoon of onion powder 1 teaspoon of parsley, dry .25 tsp paprika 7 tbsp olive oil extra-virgin – 4 tbsp. mayonnaise 3 tablespoons dijon mustard 1 tsp Tabasco sauce,.25 cup hot sauce
4 tablespoons of keto ranch dressing Blue cheese dressing is an optional ingredient. 2 tbsp vinaigrette
2 cans (15 oz each) of tomato sauce a 6 oz. jar of

tomato paste

1 tablespoon pesto; 14.5
ounces chicken broth
Chicken or beef broth may
be used to thin the sauce.

DAIRY DAIRY DAIRY
DAIRY DAIRY DAIRY
DAIRY

1 egg + 3 oz. Feta a 3 oz.
block of bleu cheese

10 ounces cream cheese
1.25 cup sour cream, 4
tablespoons butter 1 cup
(cream)

MEATS

3 slices sliced bacon 4
slices bacon cured with
hickory
3 lb. pork shoulder/butt
roast Pork chops, thick-cut
4.4 pound of chuck steak 1
pound of lean ground meat

cooked chicken, 2 cups
– 4 skinless and boneless
chicken breast halves – 1
pound boneless chicken
thighs with skins

1 cup broth de poulet de
poulet de poulet de poulet
de poulet de
2 tbsp chicken broth
(homemade/organic) 2 CUP
OF BEEF STOCK
VEGGIES
a stem of celery 3 cups
carrots, 3 cups cauliflower
6 dark leafy greens – 2 cups
Minced garlic cloves – 4-6
cloves 8 oz. slices of
mushrooms

2 minced garlic cloves -.33 cup green onion

FRUITS 1 tbsp. parsley, chopped 1 tblsp. of lemon juice CONDIMENTS

3 tbsp. kosher salt

if desired, black pepper

1-2 tablespoons Hawaiian black lava salt 1 tblsp. minced garlic

1 teaspoon of garlic salt 1 tblsp. of Italian herbs

2 tblsp. dried basil 3 tablespoons dried parsley .25 tsp paprika

.5 teaspoon of crushed red pepper flakes

1 cup red wine.33 cup water or dry white wine 5 oz. (+) coconut oil 2 tablespoons (tbsp.)
Optional: 2 tbsp. hickory liquid smoke

COOKERY

- - - - - - - - - - -

2 tbsp. coconut flour 25 cup coconut flour

Appetizer and Snack Options (Chapter 6)

DAIRY

6 eggs (large). 4 oz. cheddar

a 4 oz. container of cream cheese

3 oz. Parmesan cheese, shredded mozzarella,.25 cup

MEATS 12 slices 4 oz. cold cured salmon .5 pound of large shrimp 6 ounces. shreddable chicken

1 cup chicken breasts that have been precooked 4 pieces salami VEGGIES

1 cucumber,.25 cup celery, 3 garlic cloves a quarter cup of chopped pecans

2 tbsp. scallions, chopped (green and white portions) FRUITS

1 tsp. grated lemon zest

CONDIMENTS

1 tsp. Himalayan pink salt and 1 tsp. black pepper .25 teaspoon cayenne – 4 tbsp. barbeque sauce 1 teaspoon dijon mustard 4 tbsp. of tomato sauce 3 tbsp. mayonnaise Marinara sauce (.25 cup) .25 cup of olive oil COOKERY

3 tablespoons of psyllium husk powder 1-2 pinches pepper and salt 1.5 teaspoons of Italian seasoning

Meal Routine for a Week

Here's your seven-day food plan, complete with total net carbohydrates for each meal component. Each one is based on the ketogenic diet's daily carbohydrate allowance of 20-50 grams. You are free to have as many snacks or sweets as you like as long as you stay below your carbohydrate limits.

It's entirely up to you whatever intermittent fasting strategy you choose to spend these net carbohydrates according to the approach you pick. Always keep in mind that the ketogenic diet is very adaptable.

On the first day,

Cream Cheese Eggs (three) for breakfast
Smoked Salmon and Cream Cheese Roll-Ups for a Mid-Morning Snack – NoCook: 3rd meal: Dinner: Stuffed Pork Chops: 1 Caprese Salad: 4.6 Chicken Nuggets: 2 Cauliflower Mac and Cheese: 7

20.6 Net Carbs on Day 1 2 Biscuits and Gravy for Breakfast on Day 2
Lunch: BBQ Chicken Pizza (6.5) Mid-Morning Snack: Pizza Bites (2.8).

1.1 King-Sized Keto Salad: 9 Day Dinner: Luau Pork with Cauli Rice:

Day 3: Total carbs: 21.4 net carbs Day 2: Total carbs: 21.4 net carbs Day 2: Total carbs: 21.4

3.3 Full Herbed 'Fatty' Omelet for Breakfast

Lunch: Instant Pot Beef Chili with No Beans (Serves 8) Dinner: Instant Pot Beef Chili with No Beans (Serves 8) 2 Buffalo Beef Barbacoa – Instant Pot Day 3 Totals: 16.3 Net Carbs Cauliflower Bites: 3

Day 4: Breakfast: Bacon-Spinach-Avocado-Egg Wrap: 4
Dinner: Greens and Creamy Chicken: 2.6 Lunch: Tuna Salad: 6 Zesty Shrimp: 2.5

Day 4 totals: 15.1 net carbs, Day 5 totals: 15.1 net carbs, Day 6 totals: 15.1 net carbs, Day 7

Breakfast: Cream Cheese Eggs: 3 Lunch: Vegetarian Club: 4.8 Dinner: Garlic & Parsley Chicken Breast: 3.1 Chopped Greek Salad: 2 Snack or Dessert: Cucumber Bites & Chicken-Pecan Salad – No Cook:

Total Carbs on Day 5: 15.9 Day 6: Bacon, spinach, avocado, and an egg for breakfast. Lunch: Creamy Chicken Soup (four wraps): two

Dinner: Hamburger Stroganoff (6.1 points) and Kale Salad (three points).

Day 6 totals: 15.1 net carbs, Day 7 totals: 15.1 net carbs, Day 8 totals: 15.1 net carbs, Day 9

Blueberry Ricotta Pancakes: 6 Blueberry Ricotta Pancakes: 6 Breakfast: Breakfast: Breakfast: Breakfast: Breakfast: Breakfast: Breakfast: Breakfast: Breakfast: Breakfast: Breakfast: Breakfast: Breakfast: Breakfast: Breakfast: Breakfast: Breakfast

Cobb Salad (3 servings) for lunch

Slow Cooker Chuck Steak Dinner: 2 Day 7 Totals: 14.6 Net Carbs 3.6 Asparagus & Garlic: 2 You now have a meal plan and know what ingredients you'll need to stock up on for the next week.

Chapter 8: Tips & Suggestions

This section will help you understand how quickly you can adjust to each of the intermittent fasting and keto diet plan strategies. Don't give up; you'll get there eventually!

Using the Combo, Regain Your Confidence

Take It Cautiously: If you've never gone more than a few hours without eating, start slowly by spending 10 hours without eating and gradually increase your tolerance. It's crucial to take things slowly because if you have a lot of setbacks early on, convincing your brain to adopt a pro-fasting perspective will be more difficult in the long run. Once you start seeing actual weight reduction results, you'll find it simpler to stick with it. All you have to do now is get to that point, and everything will fall into place.

Be Aware Of Your Body's Reaction: While you should keep an eye on how your body reacts to intermittent fasting as long as you're withholding calories on a regular basis, this is particularly crucial during the first month as your body adjusts to a new manner of getting calories. While fasting might make you feel dizzy, lightheaded, shaky, irritated, furious, or weak for up to a month, symptoms that last longer are a clue that something isn't right. It's critical to be in tune with your body enough to recognize when it's time to seek medical advice.

Keep it Real: It's crucial not to hold out for immediate results. Remember, a pound of fat is equivalent to 3,500 calories not eaten. If you're feeling disheartened by your lack of progress, remember that gaining the weight you're attempting to reduce takes longer than a month or two. All that is required is patience and a genuine effort on your part.

Be Honest with Yourself: Just because intermittent fasting may provide the health advantages you want doesn't guarantee it's the best choice for you. Even if you can get through one or two fasts without difficulty, you must consider if your internal and external elements will really line in such a manner that intermittent fasting on a regular basis will be a practical option.

Consider your level of discipline, your eating habits, and your overall health. If you're searching for a means to get started on a healthy road for the first time, something with a more ambiguous failure condition could be the way to go. Remember that it's far simpler to be realistic about your chances of success and decide to go elsewhere before you start fasting in earnest than it is to struggle and fail at fasting after a week or more of serious effort.

Drink a Gallon of Water Every Day: This doesn't just mean being hydrated, which is always a good idea; it also involves drinking at least a gallon of water every day. It will make you feel full while also ensuring that your body continues to handle toxins regularly, even if it is retaining all of its fat as a result of the change. Because around 40% of individuals are somewhat dehydrated, this is a beneficial workout for the majority of people. If you don't take care of your thirst, you'll get dehydrated.

Staying hydrated can help you feel fuller for longer in two ways.

Expect Weight Loss to Be Intermittent: Every diet will experience weight loss plateaus at some point. This is an unavoidable aspect of weight loss. Weight loss will eventually resume if you maintain your consistency. Changing things up to get weight loss back on track is the worst thing you can do because it will only make it more difficult for your body to start losing weight again.

Make No Excuses: It's critical that you don't put off starting an intermittent fasting plan. Only you can ensure that you are sufficiently motivated to make periodic fasting work. Don't be afraid to put your money where your mouth is. Keep your weight-loss targets in mind.

Plan to Stay Busy: This is a good idea for the final few hours of your fast in general, but it's especially important during your transition period. Having nothing to do for several hours until you can eat again is a sure way to put your untrained body in a position where it can't help but fail. Do not fall victim to this. Simply ensure that your fast ends after a period of intense mental activity, and the last few hours will pass much more quickly.

Drinking black coffee or a zero-calorie beverage every three to four hours can help you get through the new fasts, especially when you're first training your body to expect food less often.

Caffeine is known to actively suppress the appetite, so it can help you get through the new fasts. It's crucial not to overextend yourself. However, when consumed in large quantities, many artificial sweeteners have been linked to health issues. Furthermore, it's critical not to become so reliant on caffeine that your body fails to adjust to the fasting schedule. Keep your caffeine intake under control because you don't want your body to develop a new 'bad' habit, just as you don't want your appetite to be suppressed by caffeine.

Make a Fasting Schedule. Keep in Mind: When it comes to fueling your body and mind, it's critical to consider when they're at their best. Each day should begin with the most difficult task you have to complete, as it will only become more difficult as the day progresses. Once the fasting period begins, your body will begin to naturally slow down in order to conserve energy. To ensure success, be aware of what you're up against and your limitations.

Take a Break: When you're first starting out, it's important to recognize that the transition period can be difficult, and that it will be more difficult for some people than for others. As a result, it's a good idea to begin the transition at a time when you're not under a lot of pressure or have a lot of other things going on. Anything else on your plate will almost certainly suffer as a result of your inability to make the change. "Forewarned is forearmed," as the saying goes, and planning for the change will make it easier to deal with.

How to Create Lifelong Habits

You may not realize you've lost weight at first. It's possible that you won't notice the changes for days or weeks, but the best method is to take it slowly. You're changing your way of life and letting go of old habits.

You must keep your cool.

There are no quick fixes when it comes to losing weight. The beginning of a long-term trial is difficult, just like any new challenge. You'll wonder why you waited so long to try the ketogenic diet in conjunction with your preferred intermittent fasting plan.

Make sure you get plenty of sleep and aren't stressed out.

Even before you start a diet plan, if you suffer from sleep deprivation, you will realize how stressful everyday life can be. You might think it's too late, but it isn't. Your diet will work, but you may need to make a few tweaks.

Cortisol, or the stress hormone, will rise as a result of chronic stress. Hunger levels rise as a result of that action. You end up eating more and gaining weight as a result. Whether it's decluttering your home or taking a vacation, it's important to find ways to relieve stress.

Early in the afternoon, avoid coffee and other forms of caffeine, and don't drink alcohol for at least three hours before going to bed. Alcohol can also affect the quality of your sleep, which is why you may feel tired the next day after a night out at the clubs.

Compatibility of Your Medications

It's critical to let your doctor know about your weight-loss plans. He or she might prescribe weight-gaining medications.
Your insulin may obstruct weight loss if you are taking high-dose insulin injections. You can significantly reduce your insulin requirement by eating fewer carbohydrates. Before making any changes, check with your healthcare provider again.
Other Potentially Weight-Ggaining Medications to Be Aware Of: Contraceptives that are taken by mouth
Anti-Depressants Drugs that treat epilepsy
Medication for blood pressure Medications for allergies Antibiotics

If you enjoy working out for your health, do so at least four hours before going to bed. Ascertain that your room is dark enough. You'll wake up feeling revitalized and ready to tackle your delicious keto breakfast.

Recognize the Significance of Your Cravings What You've Been Hungry For What Your Body Requires and How to Get It

Bread, Pasta, and Chocolate are all examples of carbs.

Meat with a high nitrogen content and a high protein content (nitrogen high protein meat)
Chromium Magnesium Cheese & Broccoli Nuts & Seeds of Spinach
Foods High in Salt Cheese Oil & Fatty Foods and Silicon Nuts
Chloride Fish rich in calcium Cheese, broccoli, and spinach

Added Sugars Phosphorus Tryptophan Sulfur Liver, Cheese, Lamb Eggs, Beef, Chicken Broccoli, and Cauliflower Phosphorus Tryptophan Sulfur Liver, Cheese, Lamb Eggs, Beef, Chicken Broccoli, and Cauliflower Phosphorus Trypto

Substitute high-carb foods for low-carb options.
Making a few changes to your current kitchen stock can make keeping those carbs at bay a lot easier. Take a look at the following suggestions:

Tortillas: Prepare to say no to this one, which comes in at 98 grams per serving. Enjoy a lettuce leaf instead, which contains about 1 gram of protein per serving. The 'healthy' crunch will still be present.

For 1/4 cup of almond flour, there are 3 grams of carbs. While coconut flour has 6 grams, regular wheat flour has 24 grams, which is a lot. This is why it isn't included in your diet!

Crushed pork rinds can be used in place of regular breadcrumbs if you want to keep the crunchiness. The pork rinds have no carbs, which is great news. Enjoy better fats the next time. Zucchini can be used to replace pasta. To cover your plate, use a spiralizer to create long ribbons. It goes well with a variety of dishes when prepared in this manner.

Cauliflower Rice: Instead of white or brown rice, use cauliflower rice as a substitute. 1 cup of cauliflower rice contains 45 grams of carbs, whereas 1 cup of cauliflower rice contains 2.5

grams.

Regular bowls of mashed potatoes aren't necessary.

mashed potatoes in the traditional manner Instead, eat some cauliflower mashed potatoes.
Maintain Ketosis with Snacks
Always keep a supply of high-quality snacks on hand in case your resistance wanes. Choose low-carb snacks to avoid disrupting your ketone levels. Pick a few from the list below if you have a busy schedule, but remember to keep track of your carbs.

Iced Coffee: Omit the sugar and only use full-fat milk or cream in your iced coffee. Add a pinch of chocolate, vanilla, or unflavored MCT oil powder.

Choose full-fat string cheese with no added fillers. Purchase full-fat versions of Laughing Cow Cheese Wheels and real cheese whenever possible.

Sugar added to beef jerky should be avoided. Select those that have only a few extra ingredients.

Replace chips and crackers with pork rinds. Pork Clouds, for example, is a higher-quality product that contains less offensive oil.

Pepperoni Slices: Serve with a high-fat cheese, but keep in mind that this is a highly processed product. If possible, limit the amount of hormone-free or organic meat you consume.

Snacks made from seaweed: Check the labels to make sure they don't have a lot of oil in them. Cacao Nibs: Cacao Nibs are a good substitute for chocolate chips because they have the same crunch.

If you're not using stevia, make sure your dark chocolate has a cocoa content of at least 80% or higher. Popsicles or sugar-free Jell-O: You can buy it already made or make it yourself.

Dining Out Responsibly

Before you go out to dinner, make a plan ahead of time. Prior to leaving the house, do some research. Many restaurants now have an online presence, making it much easier to eat while in ketosis. It will become more natural as you continue your preplanning, and you will be able to branch out to other locations with your newfound knowledge.

Rules of the Table

Grain, potato, and sugar are the foods that should be avoided at all costs. Vegetables, fats, and proteins should all be prioritized. Make a reservation at a restaurant that serves a nutritious menu.

Salad bar, seafood spreads, carving stations, and vegetable platters are just a few of the options available. Butter, olive oil, sour cream, and cheese are usually available in large quantities. Make the plate smaller. Fill a small plate instead of a bigger one as a mental exercise. It's worth a shot; it's effective.

Don't rush. Spend time with a friend or family member and listen to their conversation. Sip your tea or coffee while drinking water. Take pleasure in it and be content!

Remove all starches from the equation: To replace the starch, add additional vegetables or a salad. Choose a lettuce wrap over a bun for your burger or sandwich. Fats that are good for you:

Toss the meat or vegetables with extra butter.
Order a salad and a vinegar or olive oil dressing to drizzle over the meat.

You can always keep a bottle of tasty oil on hand to ensure that you have the right combination and stay in ketosis.

Drink Wisely: Water, tea, coffee, or sparkling water are the best options. Another excellent choice is decaf coffee or herbal tea. If you're craving something alcoholic, go for a dry wine, champagne, or a light beer. Also,

Consider spirits, either straight or spiked with club soda.

Condiments and Sauces to Be Aware Of:

When it comes to gravies, you can make healthier choices, but keep in mind that ketchup is primarily a carbohydrate. Keep an eye out for sauces with a high fat content, such as 'Bearnaise'. Desserts to Consider:

If you still feel hungry, try another cup of tea or a cheese platter. Serve with heavy cream and a portion of berries. How about a dollop of cream in your latte?

Here are some additional suggestions that may be useful:

Breakfast Suggestions: If you want to play it safe, nothing beats eggs. You may be off on some of the counts, but after trying a few of the recipes in this book, you'll be able to assess your eating habits for the most important meal of the day.
Suggestions for lunchtime include chicken and fish.

Diet-friendly menus are now available at many restaurants. Choose between a chicken or regular salad. Only be wary of the dressing you're using. Vinaigrette or plain vinegar are both good options.

Dinner Suggestions: Always serve your main course with a fresh green vegetable and a lean cut of meat. Try a hamburger without the bun or a tempting broccoli and steak entrée. Tasty!

Wheat products are extremely high in carbohydrates. A pita or tortilla, a baked potato, or a plate of French fries will be eliminated as a result. Request a different side dish as a substitute. Most restaurants will gladly accommodate your request, particularly if they are aware that you are on a special diet.

Restaurants that serve fast food

Even when dining out, you can have fun with your friends and family. These are just a few ways to enjoy yourself without risking losing your ketosis status. The net carbohydrate content of each of these examples is shown. Despite the fact that the Cracker Barrel restaurant specializes in breakfast foods, it also has a fantastic keto menu, which includes items such as:

7 g (+) dressing for grilled steak salad

4 g (+) carbs in side orders from grilled roast beef .5 pound Bacon Cheeseburger with 3 g (+) carbs from sides

7 g (+) dressing for grilled steak salad The following are some of the delectable side dishes:

Green Beans - 2 g Buttermilk Ranch - 1 g Blue Cheese - 2 g Spicy pork rinds - 1 g

Panera Bread is a chain of restaurants in the United States
The shop's name is unimportant. There are a plethora of keto-friendly foods to choose from. Consider the following breakfast options:
3 g Egg Bowl with Steak for a Power Breakfast
4 g Roasted Turkey and Power Breakfast Egg White Bowl Consider these menus for lunch or dinner:

Lettuce Wraps with Power Steak (6 g) Chicken Power - 7 g
7 g Roasted Turkey Bowl from the Mediterranean -

Bojangles

Simply enjoy the Grilled Chicken Salad if you want the best salad ever (net carbs - 6 grams). A small plate of roasted chicken bites is also available (4 grams). Chicken legs typically contain 4 grams of net carbs per serving. As much breading as possible should be scraped away. Toppings for a salad or dipping can be found here:

-2 g Ranch -2 g Mayonnaise 1 g Hot Sauce 0 g Bleu Cheese

Green beans, with 5 g net carbs, are the only low-carb option at the moment.

Queen of Dairy

This popular fast food chain is known for its hot dogs and hamburgers, but it also offers a variety of low-carb options. If you remove the bun from the burger, each slice will contain only 2-3 net carbs. One of the following sauces can be added to the mix:

Marzetti Balsamic Vinaigrette - 4 g Marzetti Ranch Dressing - 2 g Wild Buffalo Dipping Sauce -1 g Ranch Dipping Sauce -5 g

For a total of 7 grams net carbs, select the Grilled Chicken BLT salad option. You can also make a zero-carb breakfast by using sausage, ham, or bacon from the breakfast sides.

Wendy's

There are a few options, but these low-carb options are worth considering:

omit the bun - 4 g Double Stack - 2 g Grilled Chicken Sandwich - 5 g

Arby's offers a Chopped Farmhouse Salad (6 g) with a dressing of your choice. Choose a Meat Mountain that doesn't come with a bun or chicken tenders (6 g). Make the decision to forego the bun and make sure to account for the carbs in the dipping sauces. A few examples are as follows:

2 g (ranch)

2 g Balsamic Vinaigrette - 2 g Buttermilk Ranch - 2 g Buffalo - 2 g Light Italian - 2 g

Don't order on the spur of the moment!

Waffle House – Denny's – I-HOP

If you're going to a restaurant where breakfast is served all day, like the one mentioned above, you might want to make your own. Denny's, for instance, provides

a 'Build Your Own Grand Slam' where you can save money on bacon and eggs. To make your own keto meal, combine a few of these ingredients: Eggs

Bacon sausage Broccoli Avocado Spinach Spinach

Other/Pizza Hut/Papa John's

If you choose chicken wings, make sure to inquire ahead of time about the breading, as it may interfere with your ketosis. As examples, consider the following:

Domino's Pizza:

No-sauce wings (1 g per 2 wings) 2 g buffalo wings

1 g garlic parmesan for 2 wings at Pizza Hut 0 g for 2 wings, All-American

Dining in Ketosis: Unusual Cuisines

Food from Asia

When eating at a Chinese, Japanese, or Vietnamese restaurant, you should be cautious.

as well as Thai cuisine Maintain your concentration and avoid ordering any sweet or battered items. You should be able to order a dish with brown sauce if you ask your waiter for confirmation. Low-carb vegetables, seafood, and meat curries and stir-fries are all good options (no rice).

To add more fat to your diet, ask for butter or coconut oil. Another good option is peanut butter, olive oil, or sesame seeds. Ask the waiter/waitress for the available options.

Enjoy your dinner meal with some crispy Duck. Be sure you do not use the sweet sauce. The same non-sweet logic applies to Chop Suey with no thickeners in the sauce, when possible. Shirataki noodles are a great lowcarbohydrate choice if it's on the menu.

Mexican Cuisine

This choice of options is fantastic but leave out the tortilla chips. Order a burrito bowl, fajita

veggies, pork carnitas, chicken, and steak. Don't eat the rice and eat tiny portions of beans. Load up on meat, cheese, sour cream, guacamole, and salsa. In most restaurants, you can order double servings for these fixings at a small extra charge. You can also remove the wrapper from the burrito and eat the stuffing with a fork. Throw away the tortilla.

Indian Cuisine

Indian cuisine is another delicious option for low-carb eaters. Ask for ghee/

clarified butter, which is an Indian staple made from pure fat. You can add it to any dish. You can also enjoy Indian homemade cheese, but remember to watch out for hidden carbs.
Thickeners and flour fixings are notorious for the hiding carbs. Ask your waiter/waitress about the preparation methods. Choose curries without potatoes, kebabs, and tandoori dishes. Maybe, try some meat in creamy sauces such as tikka masala and butter chicken for a change. Avoid the portions including the naan and rice. Instead, request some Raita which is a creamy dip made from plain yogurt. It can be full-fat and served with some shredded cucumbers.

Tips for Traveling On-The-Road\sGrocery Stores

You can choose a snack if you are fortunate enough to locate a grocery store in the path of your travels. Here are some options you can quickly prepare to carry in your car:

Hard-boiled eggs Meat & cheese packs
Packaged or canned tuna Parmesan Crisps Prepackaged salads
Raw green veggies (+) dip

Whole Foods/Trader Joes

These two stores have a broader range of low-carbohydrate foods. You can choose from:

Long-aged cheese Parsnip chips

Artisan smoked meats Zoodles

Riced broccoli Riced cauliflower Seaweed snacks

Specialty sauces/condiments

Many more items are available including a wide selection of cheese and meats in the deli department.

Convenience Stores & Gas Stations

If you are on the road with limited options for dining, try some of these items for a lower

carbohydrate choice:\sDeli meat String cheese
Hard-boiled eggs Pork rinds Almonds

As you travel, you will be dependent on other people to cook for you or need to grab food on the go such as from the above choices. This convenience can sometimes pose an issue. These are some suggestions that might apply to your situation:

Add MCT Oil: Use one or two servings of the oil in your tea or similar drink prior to noon to keep your beta hydroxyl butyrate high. This is what will retain you in ketosis.

Watch Out For The Carbs: Stay away from bread, pasta, and baked goods. They will be tempting if you are away from home. If you slip and have a tasty treat that isn't in your plan, just test with a Ketostix kit and get back in gear.

Tricks to Success

While intermittent fasting is undeniably beneficial, it can be challenging to get started or to see through to the point where your body adapts to a new schedule. The following tips and tricks can help set you on the path to success.

Be Sure the Plan is for You: Intermittent fasting has a wide variety of proven benefits, but it is not for everyone. Before you attempt a fast, it is essential to have a real dialogue with yourself. Consider your level of self-discipline, your general lifestyle, your current attachment to food, any regular activities that would make fasting difficult or awkward, and your level of exercise.

Deciding to try a different fitness regime is a lot easier on day one, than after struggling through a week or more of faulty fasting.

Get Off to the Right Start "Fast": At the start of your fast, your body will still have the most fuel in its system to work with, which is why it is best to start each fast with the most challenging items on your to-do list. As you move farther and farther from the last period of time, and you take in fresh calories, your thought processes will naturally begin to slow in your body's effort to save energy. Difficult tasks will inherently seem more natural when your body is working at maximum efficiency.

Begin Your Day Hydrated: Often, the signals for hunger and the signs of thirst can get crossed in your brain. After it has sent out enough ignored thirst signals, it starts sending out hunger signals instead. As such, starting the morning off by drinking at least half a liter of water is an excellent way to quench your body's thirst from the past seven or eight hours. It should be enough to keep you feeling full for at least a few extra hours each morning. Not only will water help you feel full throughout your fast, staying hydrated is akin to staying healthy. Aim for at least a gallon of water per day.

When you're Hungry: Consider the difference between head hunger and body hunger. As you get

used to the process of intermittent fasting, you will become acquainted with several different types of hunger and ultimately learn how to tell when you are 'truly' hungry as opposed to just habitually used to eating. While it will initially be difficult to tell the difference, you will come to know them both intimately in time.

No Excuses: Intermittent fasting works on the principle that eating fewer calories than you burn is a surefire way to lose weight. This theory falls apart if you use the fact that you are fasting as an excuse to eat nothing but junk food when you are eating. Self-control and self-discipline are both equally important when it comes to eating correctly. Intermittent fasting has a wide variety of health benefits. Why not accentuate them even more with a healthy diet to go along with it? Pay Attention To Your Body Talk: While it is essential to keep tabs on how your body is responding to intermittent fasting, it is doubly important to monitor your vitals during the preliminary phase when your body is adjusting to the new feeding times. Some discomfort is to be expected for the first three to four weeks, but anything longer or more severe should be discussed with a doctor as soon as possible.

Set Lower Goals: Start Slowly: If you find that you are having difficulty starting the transition to an intermittent fasting program full bore, try moving your breakfast time back one hour each week. Before you know it, you'll have reached a 16:8 or 14:10 split without even trying.
Ups & Downs: While your body adjusts to intermittent fasting, there will be times where you are losing weight and times where your body is trying to hold on to every calorie it has. This is natural and to be expected as your body realigns its hormone levels.

Make The Fasting Time Work For You: Intermittent fasting can work around any type of schedule which is part of what makes it so great. If you find yourself feeling trapped by the period of time you are allowing yourself to eat, why don't you move it? Fasting should be about adding freedom to your schedule not restraining it.

Consume Sufficient Amounts Of Protein: There is nothing better at combating hunger than protein, plain and simple. It is also great for building lean muscle. If you find yourself unable to get through even 10 hours without eating, then it might be a sign that you should add more protein to your diet.

Go Slow – Not Fast: Even if you think you feel okay when you first begin an intermittent fasting cycle, it is always crucial to give your body the time it needs to recover. Never go more than two days out of a week without eating. There is an essential distinction between fasting and starving yourself.

Distract Yourself: Distraction is necessary as your body is adapting to your new eating habits and becomes increasingly important the farther into a fast you go. Try going out and being active when you are struggling with the plan to help refocus your thinking patterns. Besides, the exercise also helps push away the pounds.

While the preceding chapters have done their best to describe the benefits and risks of intermittent fasting, a few doubts will always arise.

Before deciding whether or not intermittent fasting is the correct option for you right now, think about the following commonly asked questions.

Is fasting going to make me sicker?

There's no reason why intermittent fasting should ever have a negative impact on your health if you maintain a nutritious diet that accounts for the vitamins and minerals you're missing out on throughout your fasting phase. In fact, some research suggests that when the body goes into fasting mode, it becomes more primed and disease resistant.

What am I going to do if I don't have breakfast in the morning?

The first thing to remember if you wake up feeling really hungry is that most of your hunger is emotional rather than bodily. You should notice a significant softening when you've completed the switch. That being stated, it's critical to drink a liter of water first thing in the morning. If you're still hungry, finish your previous day's meal with some additional protein and healthy fats, which should keep you satisfied until the next meal.

Is there a way to know whether a fasting method is right for me?

While there is no foolproof method to tell whether a style of fasting is good for you, the strongest signs are often how hungry you feel at the conclusion of the fasting period and how much energy you have after the fasting phase has begun. What it boils down to is that if you don't notice much of anything after a month of intermittent fasting, you could have found your solution.

What are the differences between the ketogenic, low-carb, Adkins, and Paleo diets?

Carbohydrate consumption is limited to 5% of total caloric intake on the Keto Diet, but low-carb diet programs have no such restriction. The ketogenic diet consists of a high-fat, low-carbohydrate diet with moderate protein. The diet causes your body to burn fat for energy because of its carbohydrate restrictions (ketosis).

The Atkins diet is first set at 15-30 grams of carbohydrates per day to encourage fat burning rather than the use of glycogen as a source of energy. Its popularity plummeted as people began to gain weight, get ill, and have their blood lipid profile worsen.

The Paleo diet is a more recent fad that encourages people to eat as our forefathers did 10,000 years ago. Because meat supplies were not always accessible everyday, it included consuming more fruits and vegetables. Fiber, omega-3 fatty acids, vitamins, and minerals are all higher in the meals. They also contained less saturated fats and less salt.

Healthy oils should provide fats in addition to meat (avocado, macadamia, walnut, olive). Refined sugar, legumes, potatoes, cereal grains, and dairy should all be included in the diet's balance.

During the week, I am able to fast effectively, but not on weekends. I'm not sure how I'm going to get this sorted out.

It's critical not to get too fixated with intermittent fasting. If you discover a 16/8 or 20/4 combination that works for you throughout the week and then allow yourself two cheat days, that's OK as long as you don't use those days to undo all of your hard work. It's all about figuring out whatever strategy works best for you and sticking with it. It's vital to focus on how effective you are every weekday rather than how successful you are on the days when you don't stay with it.

Is there anybody who wouldn't benefit from experimenting with intermittent fasting?

Anyone whose body is still developing should avoid even something as simple as a 14/10 split. Those who are still growing need as many vitamins and minerals as possible in order to reach their full potential, and even a brief fast now and again might contribute to problems later in life. In a similar vein, pregnant women should avoid intermittent fasting until after they have given birth.

What are the most effective methods for calculating ketones?

A blood ketone meter is the most accurate way to quantify ketone bodies, such as beta-hydroxybutyrate or BHB. The meter is expensive, and the materials alone may set you back about $150. It is, nevertheless, the most precise instrument.

Uriscan and Ketostix are not as accurate as other procedures for determining ketone levels in urine. Only acetoacetate levels can be measured. They're helpful at the beginning of the diet when you're simply trying to figure out how much carbohydrate you need to go into ketosis.

They are, however, easy to use, and the strips cost around $6 each month.

Acetone Breathalyzer from Ketonix: This less expensive option is used to test your acetone. Breath ketones, on the other hand, do not necessarily correspond to blood ketones in the same manner. Water consumption and alcohol consumption have an impact on them as well.

Remember that if you smell anything fruity, it's probably your ketogenic breath, which means you're in ketosis.

Ketones: How to Measure Them

Make a habit of testing at the same time each day. Concentrations are typically lower in the morning and greater in the evening. Glucose levels are greater and ketone levels are lower during periods of activity. This is why testing ketones after exercise is not recommended.

Think about how much fat you're consuming in your diet. MCTs, which are found in coconut oil, also raise your ketones. Following a high-fat meal, your ketones may have risen.

Changes in your hormone levels might cause daily swings, so don't be disheartened. This is a temporary situation.

To prevent the keto 'fruity' breath problems, drink lots of water or mint tea and consume foods high in electrolytes. Mints and chewing gum should be avoided since they may cause you to be thrown out.

ketoacidosis Keep an eye out for 'hidden' carbohydrates that might cause blood sugar problems.

Electrolytes, such as potassium, should be consumed in greater quantities. When you move to the keto eating plan, your salt and potassium levels will be reduced.

Chapter 9: A Final Note

Intermittent fasting and the ketogenic diet plan work well together to keep your energy levels stable and help you lose weight. To date, it is one of the most widely utilized performance innovations in history. Fasting may be difficult when combined with a high-carbohydrate diet. You can help reduce mood swings, poor energy, fluctuating blood sugar, and cravings by combining the two strategies. IF and Keto, on the other hand, make a fantastic partnership since they complement each other's fat- and weight-loss benefits.

You've realized that on the keto diet, you're substituting carbs with a lot of fat. Your body gets more effective at burning fat for fuel over a short period of time. You can stay in fat-burning mode all day. In summary:

Hunger Suppression: A ketogenic diet may also help you feel less hungry. The ketogenic diet permits your liver to convert fat into little energy packets known as ketones. The ketones are transported through your circulation and used as fuel by your cells. The ketones aid in the suppression of ghrelin, the body's main hunger hormone. As a result, when your ghrelin level is high, you get hungry. When you follow the keto diet, your ghrelin levels stay low even when you aren't eating. That's how you can go longer between meals without becoming hungry. When you use keto recipes, it's much simpler to fast. So start moving and relish the rewards.

No Cravings: Fat does not cause a blood sugar increase. The ketogenic diet, as you may be aware, aids with blood sugar stabilization. Individuals suffering from the affects of type 2 diabetes were able to quit taking their medication in certain situations. Fasting using keto diet programs has been shown to reduce tiredness, cravings, and mood changes that make high-carb fasting so difficult.

Fat Reduction: Keto + intermittent fasting as a fat-burning machine make a strong partnership for weight loss. Even when individuals do not intentionally reduce their calorie intake, keto methods and fasting both enhance fat loss. Because keto also lowers ghrelin, you won't be hungry or experience the emotions of deprivation that come with weight loss.

Make an Intermittent Fasting Schedule That Works: Select from a wide range of options. Every day, eat all of your meals inside an 8-hour timeframe. The following 16 hours might be fasted.

Changing your typical eating habits may be daunting at first. As a newbie, start by changing the time aspect of the specified plan as a target for the first step.

Another method to fast is to get the full advantages of fasting. You can also think about doing a water-only fast on a regular basis. You may make the procedure easier by modifying your existing meal plan to the point where you're fasting for 20 hours a day and eating your two meals in a 4-hour window. After around 30 days of this routine, you should be able to eat every 4 hours. After roughly 30 days of this pattern, switch to a day water fast that isn't as difficult. Using the ketogenic diet plan, you can produce detectable ketones:

Begin by limiting your net carbohydrate consumption. Net carbohydrates are calculated by dividing total carbs (-) fiber) by 20 to 50 grams per day, as specified on your food plan.

Protein should be limited to.5 gram per pound of body mass. (Calculate your lean body mass.) Then, deduct 100 from your body fat percentage. Calculate your current weight by multiplying that percentage by your current weight.) Replace the carbohydrates you've lost with healthy fats, aiming for 50 to 85 percent of your daily calories from fat. It is critical to get a high fiber diet, which includes vegetables. Grains and all kinds of sugar present in high-fructose fruits should be avoided. After you've reached ketosis, you'll be able to reintroduce healthy net carbohydrates (as specified in the plan).

Olives and olive oil, coconut oil, avocados, seeds, grass-fed animal products, and raw nuts like macadamia and pecans are all good sources of healthful fats. MCT oil, raw cacao butter, and 'organic-pastured' egg yolks are also excellent sources.

All trans fats and highly processed polyunsaturated vegetable oils should be avoided. Maintain your net carbohydrate, fat, and protein ratios until you've reached ketosis and your body is using fat for energy. Keto testing strips may be used to confirm whether you're in ketosis, which is defined as blood ketones of 0.5 to 3.0 mmol/L.

Just remember that when it comes to these nutritional ratios, accuracy is crucial. It's critical not to eat too many net carbohydrates. Because glucose is a more faster-burning fuel, the excess will put a stop to ketosis. Because it's very hard to properly predict the quantity of net carbohydrates, fat, and protein in any specific meal, be careful to use the recipes as directed in each meal option. Just make sure you have the necessary measurement instruments on hand. A kitchen scale, a decent set of measuring spoons, and measuring cups are all necessary.

Ketosis might take anything from 2-3 weeks to a month to acquire. Once you've determined that you're in ketosis, adhere to your plan. If you cheat and leave ketosis, it may take another month for your body to be able to burn fat effectively again. The natural advantages of cellular regeneration and rejuvenation will be maximized if you cycle "in and out" of nutritional ketosis.

Still, be aware of what is and is not healthy. Many junk items, like as potato chips and bagels, should be avoided unless they are keto friendly. Choose the healthier options, such as those listed in this advice.

Now is the time to embark on your new lifestyle plan based on your ketogenic diet. All you have to do now is choose the intermittent fasting program that best suits your requirements, and you'll be good to go!

Avoid Common Diet Pitfalls Here are a few diet-related mistakes to avoid. Making lifestyle changes doesn't have to be a chore if you prepare ahead of time for success.

You learn from your errors, and here are a few of them:

Dining by the Clock: Just because the clock reads 12:00 noon or 6:00 p.m., doesn't mean you have to eat. If you've done it before, you're aware of the danger. You should never eat until you are really hungry during dieting. Instead of looking at the clock, listen to your body.

Dieting Alone (Mistake 2): Dieting may be difficult, but many people have found that doing it alongside a friend or family member can make it seem less daunting. If everyone is on the same page, a lot of the temptations will go away. You may also join an online support group or, even better, form your own. The most important factor is to be in the company of people who understand your predicament. The Keto diet plan is all about reducing weight and inches while maintaining a healthy lifestyle!

3rd Error: Focusing Too Much on the Macros: The keto diet plan alleviates a lot of the anxiety associated with macronutrient counting. Tracking the statistics is an easy task, but avoid becoming obsessed with them.

Mistake 4: Lack of Commitment: You must be willing to alter your way of life and become committed to eating for your health. To get the desired objectives, you must fully devote yourself to the strategy. You are the only one who knows how much food you have ingested in a day. When keeping track of your food consumption, be honest with yourself.

Mistake 5: Inadequate Consumption of Essential Nutrients: Experts advise that you consume salt every day. When following the keto diet, you should drink at least two tablespoons each day, as well as Vitamin D and magnesium. Many nutrients are obtained through the meals you consume.

Mistake 6: Consuming the Wrong Fats: Seed and vegetable oils should be avoided (many stored in plastic containers). Rather, choose for saturated fats like butter, animal fats, or coconut oil, as well as monounsaturated fats like olive oil and fish oil.

Mistake #7: Eating Too Much Protein: Protein is an important macronutrient for muscle, organ, and soft tissue development. If you ingest too much protein, your attempts to attain ketosis will be thwarted. If you consume more calories than you need, the excess is converted to glucose. Mistake #8: Obsessing Over Scales: Weighing often might lead to setbacks if you don't think you're making enough progress. You must understand that the numbers on the scales represent prior work, not current work. Because your weight fluctuates everyday due to water weight, it's not as reliable as waiting a week or more to weigh.

9th Error: Comparing Yourself to Others This diet plan's success is determined by what you feel is proper and correct, not by what others say is correct. It isn't a one-size-fits-all problem; everyone gains and sheds weight differently. It doesn't make you a failure just because your buddy shed 30 pounds in 30 days when you didn't. It just implies that you must work harder and try again.

It's time for you to go off on your own.

Included is a pdf file

Keep in mind that the pdf version of this audiobook is available in your summary section. You may use it to print the recipes in this book, as well as the 7-Day Shopping List & Meal Plan.

Conclusion

I hope you liked each section of the Keto Diet & Intermittent Fasting For Beginners. I hope you found it useful and that it gave you all of the skills you need to reach your weight-loss and health-improvement objectives. Many basic ideas were offered for your ketogenic journey as you read through your new book. These are only a few of them, so remember them:

Read the labels on the foods you buy and make decisions that will keep you in ketosis.

Dinner and lunch meals should include a vegetable dish. Limit your consumption of sugarsweetened drinks and drink lots of water everyday.

It's critical to use just half the amount of salad dressing or butter that you normally would. Prepare bell pepper strips, mixed greens, and carrots as sliced vegetables. For a nutritious on-the-go option, store them in little baggies.

Only use condiments that are fat-free or low-fat.

As a snack or to accompany your dinner, include a portion of fruit. Extra nutrients are also found in the skin. Fruits that have been dried or canned are convenient and fast to prepare. Make sure they're sugar-free, however.

Frozen yogurt (fat-free or low-fat), almonds or unsalted pretzels, fresh vegetables, and unsalted plain popcorn are also good snacks.

You've already picked the intermittent fasting method you'll use on your adventure. Allow one of the programs a try and give your body some time to acclimatize. This is a new way of life, not a miraculous diet. You also know how to combine different elements to create the ideal solution for you. Making the choice to change your eating habits is a big step, and you should think about it well before taking action. If you believe you have what it takes to get the full advantages of intermittent fasting, then stop reading and begin fasting. Choose an intermittent fasting approach that appears to be a good match for you and give it a go. To begin the program, you have a large number of recipe options.

If you don't see instant results, try not to become disheartened. Make a concerted attempt to locate the one that is best for you. Above all, don't hurry; intermittent fasting is a marathon, not a sprint, and slow and steady wins the race.

The next step is to make a shopping list and go to the store to get everything you'll need to get started with your new lifestyle. Keep track of everything you eat and check the labels to make sure you're staying below the recommended limits for your fasting strategy. Some of the lessons learnt include the following:

Fast for 12-16 hours and non-consecutively fast for 2-3 days (e.g., Tuesday, Thursday, and Saturday). Fasting days should only include gentle cardio or yoga. On non-fasting days, get in more intensive exercises.

Coffee and tea are good sources of liquids (no sweeteners or milk added). Add another fasting day to your program after a two-week vacation.

Keep in mind that there is a lot more study being done on the advantages of intermittent fasting. I hope you've learned a great deal that will help you on your way to a healthy lifestyle. Please take pleasure in each step, since it is effective!

Please take a minute to leave an Amazon review of the Keto Diet And Intermittent Fasting For Beginners.

Instant Pot Salads for Lunch: Creamy Chicken Soup NoBeans Beef Chili

Cobb Salad Kale Salad Lobster Salad Tuna Salad King-Sized Keto Salad

Side Dishes for the Vegetarian Club

Garlic & Asparagus is a dish that combines the flavors of asparagus and
Buffalo Bite-Sized Cauliflower Greek Salad with Cauliflower Macaroni & Cheese

Beef is one of the most popular meats for dinner.

Burgers with Bacon and Cheese
Slow Cooker Hamburger Stroganoff – Barbacoa Beef – Instant Pot Chuck Steak

Poultry

Greens & Creamy Chicken Nuggets Chicken Breast with Garlic & Parsley

Pork

Crockpot Luau Pork Chops stuffed with Cauli Rice

Appetizer and Snack Options (Chapter 6) Snacks

No-Cook Pizza Bites with BBQ Chicken Pizza, Pecan Salad, and Cucumber Bites Zesty Shrimp
Roll-Ups with Smoked Salmon and Cream Cheese

BONUS: 7-Day Shopping List & Keto Meal Plan Tip and Suggestions (Chapter 8) Conclusion
(Chapter 9)

Description

Intermittent fasting is a new way of life that aims to maximize the nutritional value of each meal.
The concept is that you don't have to alter your diet. Simply alter your frequency of consumption
and gain a better understanding of how to prepare healthier meals. You can see real weight loss and
muscle gain in as little as one month by working with your body's natural rhythms. You won't have

to calculate your meal's carbs. All of the net carbs, protein, calories, and total fats have already been accounted for.

The following items can be found inside:

Breakfast, lunch, dinner, and snack-time recipes are among the many that will get you started on the right track. Beef, poultry, pork, and a variety of other meats are available. You'll learn a lot about the Ketogenic way of life and how to use the Intermittent Fasting Technique.

If you're still not convinced, consider the following treats you'll be missing: Blueberry Ricotta Pancakes with Biscuits & Gravy Coffee That Is Bulletproof Luau Pork with Cauli Ric Salad Chopped Greek And there's still more!

Is any of that remotely resembling a diet to you? Take a look. If that isn't enough to persuade you that a low-carb diet is effective, consider the following celebrities who have benefited from it:

Halle Berry: Halle Berry, who is 50 years old, has a figure that women half her age would envy. She attributes her good health to the ketogenic diet, which helps her manage her diabetes. "The idea is that you train your body to burn healthy fats, and so I eat healthy fats all day long," she said on a talk show in the United States.

Mick Jagger is a rock and roll legend. Mick Jagger, the lead singer of the Rolling Stones, enjoys the ketogenic diet, which may help him live longer.

Kris Jenner: Kim lost more than 50 pounds after going on a low-carb, ketogenic diet that limited her carb intake to less than 60 grams per day.

Jennifer Lopez is a well-known actress. Jennifer used to eat a vegan diet, but now she follows a mostly low-carb, keto diet plan to stay slim and toned.

Drew Carey: Back in 2010, when Drew Carey lost 100 pounds in ten months, rumors began to circulate. Was it a new magical weight-loss pill, or surgery? No. Drew's attitude toward food was actually influenced by this fact. He was eating a standard American diet, which was high in saturated fats and refined carbohydrates. Carey's results were incredible when she started eating low-carb foods.

There's no reason to hold your breath. Why not begin your journey to a healthier lifestyle right now? You already know how to add this to your own library.

CPSIA information can be obtained
at www.ICGtesting.com
Printed in the USA
BVHW051547301221
625230BV00007B/250